Birth Book #1

How to:

Be fearless in birth

Find the best doctor or midwife

Have less pain in labor

By Sarah & Steve Blight

Birth Book (this book) is not intended as medical advice (before pregnancy, during pregnancy, before birth, in birth, after birth or at any other time). *Birth Book* is for educational, entertainment and informational purposes about pregnancy and about childbirth. Always consult a qualified medical or health professional during pregnancy for anything related to you and your pregnancy or your baby's health. The ideas, comments and suggestions contained in *Birth Book* are not intended as a substitute for consulting a qualified physician during pregnancy or in birth. Nor should they ever be substituted for obtaining medical supervision regarding any activity, procedure, or suggestion that might affect your health before pregnancy, during pregnancy, before birth, in birth, after birth, or at any other time. Neither the author, contributors, nor the publishing company shall be liable or responsible for any loss, injury, or damage allegedly arising from any information or suggestion in *Birth Book*. This book may contain affiliate links. That means some links in *Birth Book* may go to websites that compensate the authors, should you decide to buy anything from those sites. If you're still reading this, holy moly, you're probably the only one who ever will in the next hundred years. Congrats—we love that you're here & have a great day!

Kudos

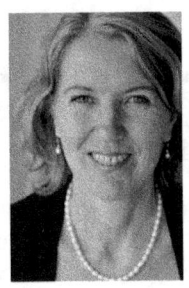

"This book will give you the crucial information and tools you need for a happy, healthy pregnancy and birth." -Dr. Sarah Buckley MD, mom of 4

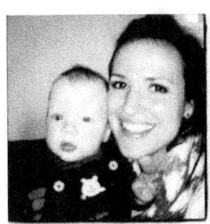

"Birth Book taught me how to feel relaxed & get through my doubts in pregnancy and in birth. This is where I started to believe that I could really do this- that what I wanted in my birth mattered and that it wasn't just a wish- it was based on proven medical evidence. Birth Book will help you have a healthier birth, whatever kind of birth you want." -Katie K., first time mom

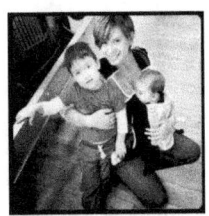

"If you're pregnant, pregnant again or thinking about trying, this book is for you! Even in my third pregnancy, Birth Book taught me things I didn't know. It has tons of valuable and practical info which is easily devoured in a few hours. And I love that it's so relaxed and different than all the other books on birth out there. It feels like you're just sitting down with these doctors and their wealth of info, as they share how to have a healthy baby and better birth. If you're expecting or know someone who is...get this book!" – Dawn S., mom of 3

Why you need to read this book ...

If you're like me... you've had at least some anxiety about being pregnant and giving birth. Sometimes that anxiety during pregnancy grows into fear and starts messing with your head. It happens in ways you wouldn't expect and goes places that can get pretty uncomfortable. You start doubting yourself. You worry (even if you've never been a worrier). And even though you know how many other moms have had babies, you still sometimes lie awake in bed thinking, "Can I really handle this?" If you're sittin' there saying, *"Yep. That's totally me."* I hear you.

We just want some direction and some answers, don't we? We want to know what to expect, so we can actually feel confident and relaxed during pregnancy and in birth. We want to know what's worked *BEST* for other moms during their pregnancy and birth, so we can have a healthier birth ourselves. We want to know how to do those pain management techniques that really work in labor. *We want encouragement.* And seriously, how about just keeping things real?

After you get done reading, you'll:

1. Know *effective techniques* to have less pain during labor and in birth. Know how to actually use these techniques in labor and in birth (even if you're getting an epidural, you'll want to know this stuff, 'cause there's pain in childbirth to varying degrees, no matter what).
2. See how strong and capable you really are! You'll feel encouraged.

3. Learn important insights and helpful tips from top doctors on finding the best doctor or midwife for you—one who believes in you, supports you and encourages you (and what they'd expect in a doctor or midwife for their own daughter's birth).
4. Learn how to have confidence and less fear from the beginning of your pregnancy through your birth.

This is the candid straightforward info I wish I had when I first got pregnant. *These are some of the topics that'll matter most to you and will help you have an easier labor and healthier birth.*

At our website YourBabyBooty.com, the top doctors and midwives, doulas, lactation consultants, fitness experts, nutritionists, other birth experts and moms open up, get real, and teach you (by video class) the most important things they've learned from helping 1,000s of moms give birth. And from their own personal experience, they teach you what they wish they knew during pregnancy and birth.

Birth Book #1 highlights four of those classes—two from doctors and two from moms totaling over 70 years of combined birth experience and nearly 5,000 births. In just a few hours of reading, you'll learn things that have taken OBs 30 years and moms, having several babies, to learn.

It's right in here for you. You can't help but be better prepared from reading this book.

It's easy and fast to read. It's written like one big relaxed conversation, like you're chattin' it up with your girlfriends. Who wants to read another stale textbook-like book about pregnancy and birth anyway? Birth Book #1 helps you avoid the stress of figuring everything out on your own. This book is for you if you want to learn how to have less fear, less pain, and be confident during pregnancy, labor and in birth.

You'll get more than just inspiration and encouragement. You'll connect with Dr. Hays, Dr. Fischbein, Kate, and Michelle, laugh with them, and hear some of their best stories and most valuable insights that will help you and your baby.

You'll also get links to the best medical research and evidence supporting what they teach. The evidence comes from the leading medical research centers in the world:

1. The US Cochrane Center at the Johns Hopkins School of Public Health (the gold standard for evidence based healthcare in the world)
2. The US Library of Medicine & National Institute of Health
3. The Journal of Perinatal Education

Birth is so much more than memorizing the signs of labor and when to go to the hospital. **It's a chance for you to meet that strong, warrior mama that you didn't even know existed. It's your chance to give birth to a new part of yourself.**

And one of the most beautiful parts of birth is that each story is as different and unique as the mama and baby in it. Our experiences, our wishes, our desires, our hopes, our expectations, our decisions are all different, and not only is that okay, that's how it really should be! There's no "one size fits all" when it comes to birthing your baby. But that doesn't mean we can't learn from each other. That doesn't mean we can't be educated on the latest research and inspired to find out what *our way* is, or stock up on the life experience of others—because one thing that's usually true: birth is full of the unexpected. The more tools we have in our birthing mama toolkit, the better. There's no right way to birth your baby, but there's a right way for you.

Whatever kind of birth you choose and wherever you decide is best to have your baby... we're here cheering you on...

"You Can Do It!"

Let's dive in & get started...

Sarah & Steve

Table of Contents

how to find a doctor or midwife who supports you, believes in you, encourages you and advocates for you.

Lesson 4   **"How To Have Less Pain In Labor (even if you're getting an epidural)" —with Michelle VanOudenallen (Mom of 2).** Learn specific techniques to have less pain in labor, relieve pressure during labor and have a faster labor. She also gives you a secret about breathing, so you can relax in labor and avoid anxiously wondering "am I doing this right?"

-Supporting medical evidence from the US Cochrane Center and the National Institute of Health

Resources &Where You Go From Here

About

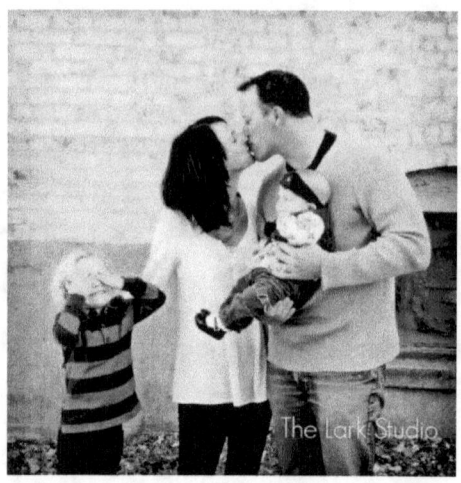

Hi, it's Sarah, we're so glad you're here! And congrats on being preggo or working on getting there.

After my first (of many) hormonal breakdowns in the middle of a baby superstore, I realized my overwhelming experience with baby registry and preparing for baby was common among new mamas. As I continued chattin' with new mamas and diving deep into the medical research and evidence on childbirth, I realized something else…that most women aren't taught and don't know how many amazing options they have during pregnancy and in birth—options that lead to easier, better and healthier outcomes for baby and mom, to feeling intensely equipped and to feeling excited about birth, rather than fearful and wanting to just "get through it." So I connected with hundreds of leading doctors, doulas, midwives, lactation consultants, fitness experts, renowned researchers, nutritionists and real moms and created a spot where they teach you these options. On the personal front, I had a hospital birth and a home birth. Both were amazing in their own way and I wouldn't trade either one! There's no right way to birth a baby, but there's a right way for you.

***

Hi, it's Steve…from my experience flying in the military, I know the value of stories. As pilots we always share and teach each other our most important "lessons learned"—the detailed accounts of each flight (good, bad, and ugly). Every pilot learns crucial information from every other pilot. That way we compound each of our experience, which helps ALL of us make better decisions when it's our turn to fly. Avoiding other's unnecessary mistakes and emulating their success is, by far, the fastest and best way to get the result you want. We've been making babies for 1,000s of years, why aren't we doing more of this during pregnancy and birth? Sarah and I decided to use this approach to help catapult you to get what you want … an easier and healthier birth.

***

You're reading one of the fruits of our labors right now. This book. If you like what you're reading, you'll love our site www.YourBabyBooty.com.

If you'd like to get an email when we release our next new book, just drop your email here: http://yourbabybooty.com/ybb/future-books

& we'll let you know when it's hot off the presses. We're working on another new book now!

Steve and Sarah have two kids: a strong willed and dare we say "spunky" 4-year-old and another "firecracker" of a daughter approaching her 2nd birthday. They live in the great state of Michigan.

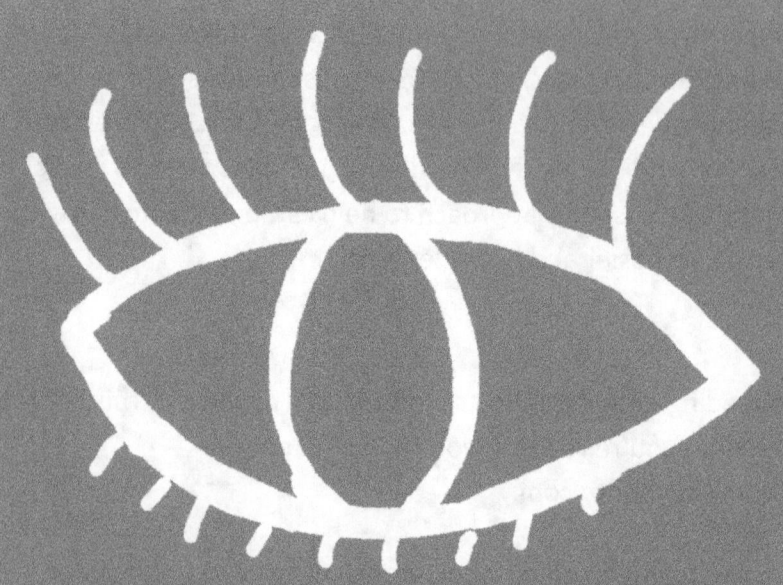

"It's a chance for women to see who they really are, not who they are programmed to be."

Dr. Bethany Hays (mom of 3, top Ob/Gyn)

"How To Be Relaxed, Calm and Confident In Birth"

–with Dr. Bethany Hays, mom of three, top OB/GYN

Sarah: What is normal birth? What does it mean, and why is it even important? To lead us through that topic is Dr. Bethany Hays. She is the mom of three boys, and a grand-mom as well, twice over. She's been an OB for over 30 years and is currently the founding practitioner member and medical director of True North, a nonprofit focusing on integrative health care, education, research, and leading other doctors and medicine into the future. Thanks so much Dr. Hays for being with us today.

Dr. Bethany Hays: Thanks for inviting me.

Sarah: You're a mom of three, grand mom, and professionally you've been catching babies for a long time. What are you most inspired to share with the expectant moms right now?

Dr. Hays: The thing I worry about most is this...the trend that we have towards surrendering the value of birthing to the control and the seduction of the medical world. I'm a person who believes in science and believes in medicine. I practice medicine.

I'm a conventional practitioner, but I think birthing is a powerful, spiritual event in a woman's life and I don't think my colleagues really understand that very well.

And so when I see women giving up their births to that medical model, I really think we're giving something important away and I would like to see more women asking the questions that maybe your subscribers are asking about, *"How should I birth my baby? What's it really like to give birth to a baby? Can I do it?"*

"Can I give birth without all that intervention and fear and risk and without surgery and without major trauma to my body?"

I would like to see that more women could find out that yes, they can do that, they can have normal births, hold their babies in their arms, have all the wonderful delicious juicy hormones running around their body when they first meet their baby, and when their spouse or partner meets that baby, and all the important things that happen when all of that comes together.

Sarah: You said you believe in science, you're a physician yourself. What place does medicine have in birth?

Dr. Hays: Well, I think the place medicine should have in birth is to catch us when we fall.

So, if we're unable for some reason to be healthy enough to have a normal birth, but we are healthy enough to get pregnant and carry the pregnancy, then I think the role of medical science is to help us complete that task, so that we have a healthy baby.

I think the role of medicine should be, and really was designed to be, used in the emergency, and not in the normal course of the event. In the same way that in our general lives, we should be learning about our bodies and how to keep them healthy, by eating right and exercising right and reducing stress and sleeping right and creating relationships that *feed* us and make us happy.

In the same way that we should be doing that throughout our lives, we should be doing that when we're pregnant, and we should be learning the physiologic process of bringing a baby into the world, which has been done for billions of years without medical science.

And, yes, babies were lost in that process, and that's where the medical science comes in, when we stumble or fall.

Sarah: You mentioned normal birth. What does that mean?

Dr. Hays: Well, that's an interesting question. Somebody said, when I was in residency training, they said, *"Have we ever seen a normal birth here at Jeff Davis Hospital?"* and we looked around at each other and we realized that normal births, we didn't actually see. Somebody said, *"Yeah, normal births are the ones that precip in the back before we get to them."*

Sarah: What does that mean, precip?

Dr. Hays: Well, they precipitate...

They deliver before we get to them "to help," you know? So, yes, there were some normal births that happened at Jeff Davis Hospital, just because we hadn't gotten there to put their IV in, and give them their drugs and give them their epidural and get them ready for their c-section and if they gave birth before we got to them, then they've had normal births.

So that was a really awakening kind of moment for me. I thought *"well, I wonder what a normal birth looks like?"*

And I think I really never saw a normal birth until I attended a home birth, until I saw what birth looks like when nobody interfered.

Then I started wondering, *"well, what would happen in my practice if I didn't interfere?"*

So I thought, *"maybe I should be doing home birth?"* Well, that wasn't going to work, because when you have MD after your name, it's very dangerous to be doing home birth. Number 1, you walk in the door and somebody's just, *"Oh, thank goodness, the doctor's here"*.

Sarah: It changes the whole mentality.

Dr. Hays: There are forceps in my hand or a knife, I mean, there's nothing I can do here that your midwife can't do, you know? So, I knew that I wouldn't get to do home birth, but I thought, well, I wonder what it would be like if I imagined that I was doing home births with each one of my patients?

And I looked into what would have happened if I had not intervened. So where did the interventions begin to produce the problems that led to the c-section or the forceps delivery or the emergency delivery?

And I really began to look at, critically, all the things that I was doing that were interventions; little things, like putting in an IV, like making a woman lie on her back in a bed, like confining her to the bed when it was time to give birth. For a while I followed women around the birthing room and there was a rumor that I did deliveries in the shower, which was not true.

I followed women around and didn't interfere with the process. If they were on the floor—and I had one woman say the floor was so wonderful, 'cause it was cool and it was solid and she felt grounded, you know? Okay, so we get down on the floor and there was a whole hoopla about that.

The nurses didn't want to get down on the floor to monitor babies, and so, instead of saying, *"We're too old to get down on the floor,"* they created this whole thing about delivering babies on the floor, it wasn't sterile.

So I went to the chief of infectious disease and I said, *"Excuse me, but, is the floor cleaner or dirtier than those mattresses that they stick the needles in after they have finished putting the IV in?"* He said, *"Probably the floor is cleaner."*

Besides that, I'm putting a sterile drape under them before I deliver them, so it's not actually delivery on the floor. They got a birthing mat. So I said, *"Okay, so it would be okay to deliver them on one of those mattresses, so if I pulled one of the mattresses off of the* stretcher, then I can deliver them on the floor?" And they said, "Uh-huh."

Really, they didn't want to get down on the floor, and I was okay, I was still young then. I probably couldn't do that now.

Or sit outside the shower room, you know, wait for signs that it was time to deliver and I learned a lot by watching what women do when you don't tell them what to do.

Sarah: So normal birth, if I'm understanding it correctly, is letting a woman go through labor and childbirth without interfering, unless she needs your help, and unless you need to intervene for the baby's health or for the mama's health. You let things just naturally progress, is that correct?

Dr. Hays: Well, that's correct. It doesn't mean you can't help the woman, and it doesn't mean you can't monitor her baby.

But it means you do as little to interfere with things that are going well as possible. You don't make a woman who's doing fine change what she's doing.

Sarah: Having a physician who knows the difference between things that are going well and things that are not going well and, when to interfere, is that an important skill?

Dr. Hays: It either takes really good training, or it takes a lot of experience in someone who's interested in your birth experience. One way I would differentiate that is when that doctor decides to come to the birth room. When does the doctor show up? If the doctor doesn't show up until you're complete and pushing, they're not interested in the process.

If the doctor shows up when you show up, they're really interested in the process. And so, a lot of doctors have an idea of when they should be present in a birthing suite or in the birth room. More importantly, it tells you something about their interest in the process of birth.

If they want to see what's going on, they're going to show up earlier. If they're showing up and sitting in the birthing room with a birthing woman through her labor, they're going to learn a lot, and those are the doctors that I would be interested in having as the person caring for my daughters-in-law and my nieces.

Sarah: A lot of times, we hear that midwives tend to be the ones who are more visible during birth, generally speaking. And that the OBs are too busy, so they're not able to be there. Is that true, in your experience?

Dr. Hays: Well, certainly—If you sit with women from two or three or four or five centimeters, throughout the rest of the labor, and it doesn't mean you're necessarily there for every contraction, but you're there as much of the time as the birthing mom needs you, or as much of the time as the nursing staff is not doing that job. Certainly if you're doing that, you're more interested in what's going on and you're going to learn more.

Sarah: A lot of times we excuse OBs, because we say, "Oh, they're really busy and they have a lot of other things they have to do. It's just not possible for them to be there," which sometimes may be

true, but in your experience is that the case? Or does it come down to being interested, or choice, or training, or just the way you've always done things?

Dr. Hays: It's true that you're not going to make as much money, 'cause you're not going to go back to the office and see as many patients while waiting for the birthing woman to give birth.

Usually if she births at night, around the weekends, you don't have that conflict, but then you have the conflict of, *"What about my own family?"* and *"How much time do I spend with them?"*

For many, many years when the phone rang at my house, there was a chorus of obscenities, which meant, *"oh darn, Mom's leaving again"*, because obviously I'd get up and go help a mom birth her baby!

Physicians are torn and then, remember a lot of people who became physicians didn't really become physicians to do birth attendance, they became physicians to do heroic things with knives and forceps and machinery and ultrasounds, and they want to learn the technology—they want to be there for the emergency.

Sarah: So why does it matter, Dr. Hays, for women to have normal birth?

Dr. Hays: Well, I think there are several reasons. Probably the most important is that when a woman goes through the process of labor and birth, she learns that she is capable of doing something that's really hard, and that is really tiring, and that is really uncomfortable.

I'll even use the P word, it's really painful. And then, if she is successful, if she is helped to be successful, and given the accolades that she deserves for getting through that process, there is nothing else in her life that will ever scare her in terms of pain, hard, long, tired.

You can go through your life going, "*Boy, this is the worst pain—oh no, this isn't that bad. Never mind. This is A-okay.*"

Or, "*Boy, I've never been this tired—okay, wait. No, I have been—okay, this isn't that bad—I can keep going,*" you know?

It's where you learn that you can keep going. And when you're raising small children, there are a lot of nights that you spend up and that you're exhausted and now, with young mothers working outside the home and then coming home and doing the second shift, and sometimes the second shift lasts all night, and then they get up and go to work again, you don't have to have some training that tells you, "*I can do this, I can get through this.*"

So I think we miss that. The other thing is that sometimes women, as they give birth, it's like there's a picture frame that goes past them, and for just a second they see themselves, the real them, and then it passes on.

And they see the person that they really are, not the one they've been programmed to be.

I used to say to husbands, "*be prepared, because the woman your wife really is, is going to show up at birth.*"

And most men are amazed at the woman who shows up, like, "*I had no idea she could do anything like this! I had no idea how powerful she is!*"

So a lot of women do it over and over again, 'cause they want to get that glimpse over and over again. But it's your opportunity to see yourself in a different light, and you don't get it really anywhere else. Men go to war to get things like that, actually I've heard husbands say, "If men did this, there wouldn't need to be any wars..."

Because this is how women learn about the importance of relationships and about doing something really hard and about getting through, and about being there for someone no matter what. Men get that in war.

They get to find out what it's like to do something really hard and protect your buddies and do something that's maybe painful and scary and life-threatening, and so—I've actually had men say "*men go to war and women go-to childbirth.*"

The trouble is that men don't get anything back, and we get a baby. We get something back for all that work and all that pain. And that's what's extraordinary about it.

It's the only thing you ever do that you get a reward for it.

Sarah: It's pain and hardship with a purpose and a wonderful gift at the end.

Dr. Hays: Wonderful reward at the end!

Sarah: So, does having a normal birth mean staying out of the hospital? Does it mean not having an OB/GYN? What does it mean, having a home birth with a midwife?

Dr. Hays: I hope it doesn't mean that, because if it does, then there are 3,000 women that I have helped to give birth who didn't have normal births, and that would make me really sad.

So, no, you can have a normal birth in a hospital if you have the *right people* with you and the *right hospital* with the *right policies*. It's really all about what do they do once you get there.

Is it easier to have a normal birth at home? Probably...for a lot of women. What we really want, what we women really want is we want to be able to choose where we give birth, and we want to be able to change our minds in case we chose wrong.

So, I've had women who, planned the home birth and then realized at some point that they needed a hospital, they didn't feel safe at home. They couldn't do it at home, and then thank goodness, they found a way to come in and be at a hospital and not be abused by the hospital, which happens a lot to home birth women who come to the hospital.

And they were always amazed when, I would come in to take care of someone who'd been laboring for three days at home, and I would sit down and watch what was going on, see what the feel of the people in the room was.

Usually it was suspicious. Like, "*What are you going to do to her?*" and I would sit with her for a while and watch her do a few contractions and then I would say, *"So tell me what you know about what's going on.* What's going on in your body?"

And that kind of diffused the whole, *"Oh my god, the doctor's going to come in and tell me what to do. No, the doctor wants to know what I know about what's going on here."* And then, of course, sometimes they would just blurt out exactly what was going on, and you'd say, *"Okay, well, let's see what we can do to fix that."*

Or…*"I'm scared." "Okay, what are you scared of? Let's talk about that. Your baby's fine, we've checked out your baby, your baby's fine."* 'Cause the first thing I'm going to do in a hospital is make sure the baby's okay, because I don't really think any of this makes any sense if you don't get the baby.

So, my number one goal was always to get a healthy baby, and then my number two goal was to have the mother and baby able to be together. I saw myself as helping to create families, and if the mother and baby get separated, then it's not as easy to do that.

And then the third goal was for the mother to get the birth she wanted. And sometimes that is not the birth that I want, so right now, tonight, I'm talking about the birth I want—I want for mothers, and one of the things I had to learn to do as an OB was to let go of that and accept that there were women who didn't want the birth that I thought was the brilliant, wonderful and beautiful birth. They didn't want that birth, and that's okay with me.

Sarah: Is there a difference, Dr. Hays, between normal birth and a natural, unmedicated childbirth- Are those the same thing or are

they different? Can you have a normal birth and have an epidural or have narcotics or have drugs?

Dr. Hays: You can have a vaginal birth, with narcotics, with an epidural, with a lot of interventions. You can have vaginal birth of a premature baby. You can have vaginal birth in a high-risk mother.

Sarah: But that's not the same thing as normal birth, what we're talking about tonight?

Dr. Hays: Well, I'm not saying that it's necessarily abnormal to get a little help. I'm just saying that there are lots of kinds of help that you can give to a young mother who's struggling in her labor. And sometimes it's just to come in and sit with her and ask what's going on.

I remember a mother who—the nurses came and said, *"Oh, she needs pain medicine,"* she was 7 cm and I went in to sit down with her and I said, *"So, let me just sit here with you for a minute and see what's going on."* She was doing Lamaze, so she was doing breathing and her husband was all energetic going, *"Breathe, breathe,* breathe," and the nurse is taking her blood pressure and monitor's going beep, beep, beep, and it was just frantic.

I mean, she was frantic. And I said, *"You know, this breathing thing... just breathe,"* I said *"In between contractions, just go somewhere else. And then when the contraction comes, we'll get through it."* And she said, *"Oh, okay."*

She was gone. And the contraction came and nothing—and she didn't come back, and then the next contraction came, and she didn't say a thing. And her husband said, *"Did her contractions* stop?" And I said, "Nope, they're still going, every three minutes." And he said, "Well, where did she go?" I said, "I don't know. We'll have to ask her when she comes back."

So, about an hour later, she opens her eyes and she says, "Ooh, I think I need to push." I said, "Okay."

So, she pushes her baby out and I said, "So, your husband and I want to know where you went." She said, "Well, I don't know, but it was really great there." I said, "Well, if you ever figure out where you went, I want to know about it," and she said, "Okay."

So she comes in for a postpartum check-up and she says, "Okay, I can tell you where I went now." I said, "Okay." She said, "You know, when you came in, everything was just frantic and the noise and my husband saying 'breathe, breathe,' and I was just, I was just crazed, and then you said 'go somewhere else,' and suddenly, I found myself in a quiet room, and everything in the room was white. And it was so peaceful.

"And then..." she says, "My favorite uncle, who died recently, showed up and he sat down with me and we chatted. And it was just great. And then the next thing I knew, I was pushing my baby out." And I said, "Wow. Who knew you could have a dead uncle as a doula."

Clearly, that's an example of how spiritual a birth can be. And, if you can connect up with something that amazing, that big, then contractions don't seem very important or strenuous or maybe even painful.

I've seen hundreds of really fascinating, amazing ways that women deal with labor, but you have to watch in order to see them, and you have to give the woman an opportunity, you have to find the key that opens the door for *that* woman. For this woman, it was just me saying, *"Go somewhere else."*

Sarah: What have your three most remarkable births been, and how did they teach you to respect birth?

Dr. Hays: Oh, let me tell you my favorite birthing stories. So, this was a woman who hired a doula, and the doula was one of the original doulas of Kennel and Klaus's Doula Study at Jeff Davis Hospital, and her name is Nadia. And Nadia spoke five languages and had lived all over the world and was the most wonderful, gentle, lovely person. Nadia would speak very softly with sort of an accent, and so she came in with this patient, and the patient was laboring away with her first baby, and she had had an epidural, because she was afraid that her husband would leave.

When she got uncomfortable, he got very nervous, and she was afraid he would leave. So, this time, she came to me because she said, *"I want to have a normal birth, and you're the person I understand does that,"* and she said, *"I had the first baby—I had an epidural for my husband, but this time, I'm having a baby for myself."* I said, *"Well, great!"*

So, Nadia came in with her and they're laboring, and every now and again, she would tense up, and Nadia would say, *"No, you're doing beautifully."* And so, Nadia gets her through the labor, and some way or another, she ended up in a bed. And she's lying, kind of on her back in the bed, and Nadia's on one side and I'm on the other and the husband is, like circulating around the edges of the room. If he could have gotten further away, he would have.

But, all of a sudden, she says, *"Oh, I think I need to push,"* and I checked her and she's complete and I said, *"Yes, you're complete now. Just listen to your body, whatever it says to do, just do that."*

Suddenly her husband—I'm going to call him Jerry—suddenly, her husband Jerry comes over to her bedside, he realizes he's going to make it through this labor, and he comes over and he reaches down and he kisses her very sweetly on the lips, and she looks at him and she says, *"Oh, Jerry, kiss me again. It feels so good when you kiss me."* And suddenly, Jerry has a job.

And he reaches down and he grasps this woman in his arms and he pulls her up and he plants what—you know, Kevin Costner called the long, slow, deep, wet kiss that lasts three days. And now, Nadia and I are kind of going, *"Oof! We're not supposed to be here!"*

And so, she's not pushing but, you know, suddenly the baby's head is crowning... and it's crowning... and it's crowning... and I look down and Nadia looks at me and they're kissing!

And the skin peels back and over the baby's forehead and the baby's eyes are kind of blinking, and then the head comes out and I said—I sort of signed to Nadia, *"I think I'm supposed to do something in here,"* and she says, *"You're the doctor, go ahead and do it!"*

So, I reached down and I gradually, very gently deliver the anterior shoulder and I slide this baby up on the mother's abdomen. Now, they're still kissing! So, all of a sudden, she looks up and she looks down and she says, *"Oh my goodness!"* She said, *"I forgot I was in a hospital!"*

Imagine what it was like for this baby to be born into love that powerful!

I would love to know what this kid turned out to be.

She went to an orgasmic place, you know, the orgasmic birth some people talk about. And after that, I started thinking, well, why doesn't everyone do this? Why doesn't every woman have a birth like this?

So every time I saw a woman who birthed without a lot of hoopla and pain and frustration, craziness, I would ask, *"Well, what were you doing? What was going on in your head?"*

And they would say things like—one woman said, *"Well, you know,"* she was a surfer, she said, *"you know, when you're surfing and the waves get really big, if you stay on the surface you get thrashed around and you get kind of—blown up against the reef and you get all cut up.*

But if when the wave comes, you just dive down and hold onto the reef and let the wave pass over you, then you can come up in between and you're fine. So, when I have a contraction, I just dive down and let it pass over me, and then I can come up in between and I'm fine."

And so, the next birth that I was with her, I'm watching her and you could barely tell she was having contractions. Her respiratory excursion would get a little deeper, and about 9 centimeters, she kind of opens one eye slowly and she looks at me and she says..."*Surf's up.*"

And then she closed her eyes and did her birth.

So I'm always on the lookout for those women, 'cause that wasn't the way my births were, you know. I got trained in Lamaze and I did breathe, breathe, breathe, breathe, breathe, until I couldn't breathe anymore, and then I screamed a lot and a baby came out.

But I got him out, you know.

Sarah: So how much of that, Dr. Hays, do you think is preparation and how much do you think of that is just like personality type or disposition as a person? Or is it kind of a melding of the two?

Dr. Hays: You know what, I think a lot of these women never hear those stories.

They never get to hear that that could happen. I had a woman who delivered at a hospital, she'd been at the hospital from 28 weeks with placenta previa. She gets to 36 weeks, they re-ultrasound her and say, "*Whoop! The placenta has moved.*"

Well, placentas don't get up and move, okay. She'd had a blood clot in the lower segment that they had mistaken for placenta. That was fine that they kept her in bed, but now they're saying, "*But your baby is in there with decreased amniotic fluid, we need to induce you.*" So, they couldn't induce her on Friday, so on Saturday she gets the go-ahead to get induced, and unfortunately it's the weekend, now the strange doctor comes in.

So I come in and sit down. I say, *"Okay, so, what do you know about having babies?"* She says, *"Nothing! They told me I was going to have a c-section."* I said, *"Okay, so we're going to do a little on the job training, but I'm going to start with some stories."*

So I told her some stories, okay? And then she went into labor—I think she had, you know, like one little tiny dose of pain medicine, and then she did a beautiful birth, and I said, *"Wow! So, aren't you the birthing woman?"*

And she said, *"Well, it was the stories."* I said, *"The stories?"* She said, *"It was the story you told me."* She said, *"I had heard that story about the white room and I thought, That's the way I want to be in birth."* And she says, *"And now, I want to be one of your stories."*

And she is!

Sarah: So for the women who are thinking, this all sounds fantastic, I want to have a normal birth. What are the three things they need to do this week to have a normal birth? Where does it start?

Dr. Hays: It starts pre-conceptually. It starts by having good nutrition, by wanting the baby, by planning the baby, by inviting that baby into your life, and then making room, making room in your house, in your body, and in your spirit to have another person in your life. Then it's good food, lots and lots and lots of preferably organic vegetables. Protein and carbohydrate balance that keeps you—not just blood sugars that pass the test, but blood sugars that are really normal.

And then it takes learning everything you can, learning and doing some work on what your stumbling block would be towards having that birth.

There's a wonderful book called, "Birthing from Within," and it really teaches young mothers to look into what their stumbling blocks might be. They journal about them, they do artwork. I'm quite certain that's how my niece got the wonderful birth that she had. She had some real discovery that went on during her pregnancy. Then it's picking the right people to be with you. Picking people to be with you, you need to find somebody to be with you who's not afraid of it.

If the people around you are afraid, you're going to be afraid. I've had women say, *"Well, I was really scared, and I looked at my husband and he was really scared, and I looked at the nurse and she looked really scared, but I looked at you, and you didn't look scared, so I just kept looking at you."*

And you have to practice as an obstetrician, you know, the 'I'm not scared, so you shouldn't be either look.' But apparently I have a very transparent face, so that if I am scared, it's bad. And one time one woman said, *"I was pretty sure my baby was dead* by the look on your face..."

But you've got to have people with you who are not afraid of birth, and not afraid of what happens to women in birth, because they can get pretty crazy. Things can get pretty wild, and you've got to be okay with that, that's normal. Every woman has her birthing place, her place where she is when she's in labor, and some of them are crazy places and some of them are quiet places and some of them are wild places. So you have to have people who are okay with that and know how to find that.

Sarah: So that would include also your doctor, hospital, or location for your birth. Obviously for everyone it's going to be different—midwife, doctor, family practice, whatever your choice is. So that also plays a role, too, not just in the actual, like, labor support, but also in your prenatal care and all that stuff. Your doctor or health care provider, that should be a consideration as well?

Dr. Hays: You need to have a plan, whether you're birthing in a hospital or birthing at home, you need to have a plan for what happens if you stumble and fall. So you need to have a plan to rescue your baby, and that plan needs to be seamless, it needs to be initiated without a lot of hoopla, they need to know you're coming; they need to have a plan for you. And you need to be trusting those people enough, that when things look scary or dangerous, you can let go and say, "*I trust these people to help me have a healthy baby.*" Then you need to have people who are with you. So, that could be your spouse, your partner, as long as your partner is willing to be with you for every contraction. That is very hard for one person to do, so I vote, have some other people there, people who know how to help you through contractions.

A doula can be great. I'm a big fan of grandmothers, provided grandmother knows how to help somebody give birth. And, you know, she doesn't have to have birthed babies herself, she can have had c sections.

My niece's mother—my sister-in-law, had three c-sections, and when she found out her daughter was planning to have a normal birth, she came to me and said, "*Teach me, quick, how to be a good doula for my daughter,*" and she was brilliant! I mean, the child got to the hospital complete. I mean, how much better can you do as a doula?

Sarah: So, what I'm hearing you saying—is that normal birth means really deciding what you want, and then putting things in place to make that possible, all the way through from the start—from conception to delivery, and you've walked us through what that looks like. Are we missing anything else?

Dr. Hays: Yeah, there are some things you're missing. One thing is something that happens to a lot of women in our culture is rape or sexual abuse. And it is one of the stumbling blocks that keep women from having normal births. If you have suffered that experience, one of the mechanisms that your brain can use to allow you to survive it is to disconnect from your body—disable.

This is not me that's getting raped, and so if you suddenly find yourself in labor getting very powerful signals from a part of your body that you maybe haven't talked to in twenty years, you're going to freeze up and have a very hard time sharing that part of your body with your baby. And so, you need to have done some work on that. And then, you know you can heal that event in birth. So instead of saying, "*Baby's not coming,*" we don't know why it's not coming down, you know, you can help a mother to feel that part of her body, to feel her baby's head.

To help her baby's head come through her pelvis, to know that she's in charge of it. She can make it happen as fast or as slow as she needs to, that it doesn't have to be a terrible trauma, as long as she's in control of it this time. And so I have sort of reprogrammed some of that information, even in birth, without ever mentioning the word rape.

But I knew that's what was going on. I prefer that women do that work in advance and maybe do some work with perineal stretching and preparation, to prevent episiotomies, so that they can heal that all the way through to claiming their body as their own, claiming that part of their body now belongs to me, because I get to choose to share it with my baby. Instead of, "I can't have any signals coming from that part of my body," so you'll have to give me yet another trauma, a major operation, to get my baby out of me. Now I've got two traumas, I've had a cut—a knife cut me open, and I've had a rape. I just don't see how that helps a woman.

Sarah: So it would be important if you've experienced that in your life to share that with your health care provider?

Dr. Hays: Not necessarily.

Sarah: Or someone who's supporting you in birth?

Dr. Hays: Go and work with a therapist around that, or find a midwife or someone who does sexual counseling who can really help you walk through that again and reclaim that part of your body. I just think that is a stumbling block that happens not infrequently, and it's not on the radar screen of most physicians.

Sarah: Are there any other stumbling blocks that you want to talk about?

Dr. Hays: Big one is nutrition.

The big one is having the right diet for your body type and stress level and exercise level. And eating enough vegetables to get all the vitamins and minerals that you need, preferably from food, but there may be some that you need in addition to that. Staying away from junk food—it's not just alcohol we need to stay away from, it's junk. We need to stay away from food that doesn't have any value, it just has calories and sugar and fat.

All of which—doesn't mean fat is bad. Good fat is good.

I have a four-part food plan for pregnant women. It's... 1) Balance protein and carbohydrates—get rid of sugar. 2) Eat five servings or more of bright colored vegetables. 3) Eat small frequent meals. And 4) Eat good fat, not bad fat.

Getting rid of sugar is part of the balancing protein and carbohydrate. And good fat, not bad fat—good fat comes from plants or cold water fish, and bad fat comes from animals and man-made fats, transfats.

Sarah: I want to thank you so much, Dr. Hays, for sharing your stories, your experience, all of your knowledge with all of the mamas and with us.

If you live in Maine, you'll definitely want to check out Dr. Hays at True North for your health care needs.

Supporting Evidence

Remember when Dr. Hays talked about not interfering in normal birth? She said, "*I learned you don't make a woman who's doing fine change what she's doing.*" The evidence says… "*unless there is a clear medical reason for an intervention, interfering with the natural process of labor and birth is not likely to be beneficial…*" The Journal of Perinatal Education[i] studied how *routine* intervention during normal labor and birth can hinder your birth (routine means procedures done when they're not medically required, ie—when a woman is doing fine).

She also talked about how the people surrounding you during labor and birth help you stay relaxed, focused, confident, and avoid feeling anxious. In birth, those people are called "continuous labor and birth support." A doula is a great example of continuous labor and birth support. They're 100% *focused on you, they serve your every physical & emotional need.*

"Kennell and Klaus" was the original study done (by Dr. Marshall Klaus & Dr. John Kennell) on continuous labor and birth support that Dr. Hays referred to. In 1967, Dr. Klaus ran the Neonatal Intensive Care Unit (NICU) at Stanford University and noticed how many parents had a *really* hard time adjusting to their new babies. Back then new moms weren't allowed to see their babies in the preemie-nursery until right before discharge (crazy huh?!?). So Dr. Klaus partnered up with Dr. Kennell to study emotional and physical bonding during birth. Their research, and proven results led to preemie babies and full-term babies "being allowed" to be with their parents right after birth. Can you imagine if you weren't allowed to see your baby after birth?

Well, guess what? They also discovered all the HUGE benefits of continuous emotional and physical support from one woman to another (that's what we call continuous labor and birth support today). Along with a few other birth experts, they named this person giving the support "Doula." Doula means "woman's servant" in ancient Greek.

A review[ii] of over 15,000 women, from the US Cochrane Center at the Johns Hopkins School of Public Health, shows women with continuous labor and birth support are more likely to go into labor naturally on their own (meaning they're not induced), request less pain medication, have shorter labors, have less chance of a c-section, have less chance of forceps or vacuum delivery, and were "more likely to be satisfied" with their births.

What's interesting... the results were best when the labor and birth support *was not* a member of the hospital staff or in the laboring mama's social circle. And compared with women who didn't have any continuous labor and birth support, women *with* continuous labor and birth support (who were not on the hospital staff or in her social circle) were:

- ✓ 28% less likely to have a c-section
- ✓ 31% less likely to get induced to speed up labor (with Pitocin)
- ✓ 34% less likely to think their childbirth experience was negative

Mamas who had some form of continuous labor and birth support (but not necessarily someone outside of the hospital staff or her social circle) also had a:

- ✓ 14% decrease in the risk of their baby being admitted to a special care nursery
- ✓ 9% decrease in pain medications use

The link to the continuous labor and birth support evidence from the Dr. Kennell & Dr. Klaus study[iii] can be found in the sources list at the end of this book.

Why does continuous labor and birth support help you have an easier & healthier birth? For several reasons.

First, your emotions control your body (the mind-body connection has long been scientifically proven—think about top athletes who train to optimize their mind-body connection for better performance). Your brain (the hypothalamus gland) releases chemical hormones (oxytocin) into your blood telling your body to relax. When you're relaxed, your body performs at its peak level and more easily does what it was designed to do (you have more efficient contractions, you feel less pain, your baby's heart rate stays regular, etc.), which is exactly why the best athletes are often the most relaxed athletes. Having someone by your side all the time, who knows birth inside and out and who knows exactly what you want (because they know your birth plan like the back of their hand), helps you stay relaxed from start all the way to finish.

Second, doulas are professionally trained and know how to help you use movement, gravity, different positions, affirmations, and other tools to help you labor most effectively. They're expert coaches in labor and birth. They guide you. They help you along through labor. They constantly encourage you. They help you find what's most comfortable for you and what works best for you.

Lastly, doulas act as a buffer between the hospital and you. That's super important because all kinds of things *will happen* in hospitals that *will distract you*, like shift changeovers for staff, lighting in the rooms or hallway, nurse personalities, smells, beeping machines, the procedures themselves, etc. **Staying focused is k-e-y**. And this might be the biggie, if your doctor wants to do a procedure that isn't medically required and that you don't want (i.e. while you're in the zone with baby), doulas will gently remind you to speak up and say *"no thanks, Doc, I don't want that."* They know how things roll, they can see things coming, they can heads things off, they've been through it many-a-time before... and through it all, they advocate for you. Are you picking up how H-U-G-E that is?! Steve was super daddy at my birth, but as amazing as he was (and still is) he didn't know what he didn't know. Ya know? Your desires for birth (you can call it a "birth plan") happening as smoothly as possible, is a doula's sole job.

Okay, here's something to think about... some hospitals have doulas on staff. And that might be a really great option for you! But it's important to remember that not all doulas are created equal (just like not all doctors or midwives are created equal). Just because "a doula" is in the room doesn't mean you'll want "that doula" in the room. Having someone new, that you've never met, "be assigned to you" while you're laboring *may* not be what you want.

By hiring your own doula, you've had time to get to know them, to trust them, to like them, to laugh with them, to share with them, to build a relationship with them. You already know for a fact they can help you relax. Just something to think through as you decide *what you want* and what's best for you.

The bottom line... the evidence shows that your continuous labor and birth support can have more of an impact on you and your entire birth than anything else. When you feel safe, secure and advocated for... you'll labor easier and you're more likely to have a healthy birth. That's why so many doctors, nurses, midwives, and moms swear by doulas.

Our friend Dawn, a mom of two and pregnant with her third baby, just said to us the other day... *"from my experience- I would say that a doula is one hundred percent the most important person to have in the room, especially for a first-time mom."*

Some insurance plans cover doulas, find out if yours does. They can range from a few hundred dollars on up.

In Short

Can you imagine your doctor or midwife joining you wherever you wanted to give birth... in the shower, in the tub, or on the floor? And doing whatever it takes to make you feel safe, comfortable, attended to, advocated for, and having your back so much that they "conversed" with other hospital staffers to get you want you want?

Can you imagine your provider quietly sitting down with you during labor and asking you what *you* knew about what's going on... then sitting there with you, helping you, soaking up the journey of birth (instead of walking in, telling you what to do, then leaving)?

I didn't.

I had no idea this relationship could even exist in the world of healthcare providers. The proof was in the pudding—the doctor I chose to catch my first baby—I asked him a question one day at one of my appointments and he told me, *"It's in that packet of information I gave you. Just read that."* The troubling thing was that I wasn't that troubled by his response until later, until I understood that that's not an okay response for anyone to give me. Not a plumber, doctor, realtor, stylist, or wedding planner, and especially not the doctor who I'm entrusting our baby's birth to (and am paying him for).

Would that rub you the wrong way? 'Cause I have a feeling I'm not alone.

Did you catch Dr. Hays' tip to ask around so you can find out if your doctor is even interested in your birth? Hint: many aren't. But some are! You want to find that out now... *before* you actually need them to catch your baby!

Thankfully, I broke up with my *"look in the packet of info"* doctor before my baby came. Because packets of info don't give you good care—people do—people who sit down and take the time to get to know you as a woman, not just an incubator for your precious cargo.

The empathy, support, and encouragement that you CAN find in a doctor or midwife, are the perfect compliments to the warrior woman you will become as you birth your baby.

I look back at my first birth and I think, *"dang, who was that woman?"* I (and my husband) experienced a side of myself I had never seen before. I was strong. I worked through my fears. I embraced the pain. I dug down into the deepest part of me and knew that the only person who could birth this baby was me. It was up to me. And I did it. There was a resolve that I never knew I had, a strength that I had never seen in myself before. Someone once asked me if I had ever run a marathon, at which point I snorted, laughed, and said *"I'm just not that tough. I would never have the stick-with-it-ness to even train to do one, much less finish a race. No way. I'm too much of a wuss."* If anyone asked me that question today, I would say, *"Heck yeah, I could do it! I can do anything!!"*

Birth is such a monumental time in a woman's life, not just because of the amazing bundle of joy who is born, but as Dr. Hays says, *"it's where we learn to keep going."* And that knowledge is powerful. It spurs us on in motherhood, because as moms we need to come back to that place a lot—we're strong... we can do it!

Okay, let's get back to doulas for a second. If you're not sure if a doula is worth the money, I know... I felt the exact same way! And Steve definitely wasn't sold on the idea. He had a completely different approach for getting an answer to the question "Is a doula *really* worth the money?" He's a logical thinker and thought about it this way:

"Okay, we're shooting for the best 'complication free, minimal intervention unless medically required, healthiest mom and healthiest baby' birth we can have. What can I do to increase the chances of that happening? Would I support a doctor giving Sarah 'a procedure' in the hospital that has been medically proven to:

1) Have zero risk and no side-effects

2) Reduce the probability of a c-section

3) Reduce the probability of delivering my baby by forceps or vacuum

4) Reduce the probability of her needing to be induced

5) Reduce pain

6) Increase her chances of going into labor naturally (which is called 'spontaneous labor')

7) Help her have a faster labor

8) Increases the chance for 'greater satisfaction' of the entire birth itself

9) Increases the chance of having a healthy baby (higher apgar score at 5 minute mark after birth)?

Yes, of course I would.

So would I support a 'non-procedure' that would give Sarah and baby all those exact same benefits? Yes, absolutely I would.

A better question... 'why wouldn't I support something that isn't even a 'procedure' at all and gives Sarah and baby all those benefits during labor and birth?'

I can't think of any reason. My family's health is my best investment. Yes, I want to hire a doula and get all those benefits that have been scientifically proven.

But can we really afford a doula? Or a better question... 'how do we make sure we can afford a doula?'

Would I rather have... a healthy wife and healthy baby or the gazillion 'cutesy' clothes and random baby things I know for a fact we don't need (that a lot of people will give us during the baby shower)? Easy answer.

So all we have to do is mention to 10-15 friends/family, before the baby shower, that we have a doula fund. We'd be grateful if they'd help us have a healthy birth by contributing for a doula, instead of buying clothes or anything else. Baby and mom's health are priority #1. Boom... our doula is paid for!"

Maybe you found Steve's way of thinking through the "is a doula worth it?" question helpful. Maybe not. Take it or leave it, whatever works for you.

*Another tip is that doulas who are training to get certified need to attend a certain number of births beforehand. There are fantastic doulas who will support laboring mamas for a fraction of their normal fee and some might even offer their support for free. You can contact DONA or Doula Trainings International to find out if there are any trainees in your area.

Okay, and the last thing to mention is something you'll use every single day and it simplifies all the confusing nutrition "stuff" you'll hear during pregnancy. Remember when Dr. Hays talked about her 4 part nutrition plan? Here's a super easy way to remember that plan—use the acronym **5 SPF** (like the sunscreen). Why are they important for you and baby:

5—**5 Servings of Bright Colored Veggies and Fruit:** Bright colored veggies and fruit are loaded with nutrients fueling your baby's growth. They also give you fiber for digestion. Dark green veggies (kale, chard, beet greens) have tons of folate. Folates are the "B vitamin that every cell in your body needs for normal growth and development" (according to the March of Dimes Foundation, who works to improve the health of babies and moms). Folates are believed to help prevent neural tube defects in your growing baby. Neural tubes are the part of your baby that turn into their brain and spinal cord- yeah, slightly important. Eat dark green veggies. Then eat more.

S—**Small meals frequently**: Your body is super busy providing everything your baby needs as he or she grows in your womb. Eating small meals frequently makes sure that your blood sugar stays stable so you can avoid getting shaky. It also helps with nausea, heartburn and can help with morning sickness. When you eat small meals frequently, you're more likely to eat healthy things since you won't turn into a ravenous wolf who will consume anything in her path... believe me, this is knowledge from personal experience. Just ask Steve.

P—Protein balance with carbs: Protein contains amino acids, which are the building blocks of your baby's cells. Proteins are crucial for baby's growth (especially in 2nd & 3rd trimester), they help with your baby's brain development and also assist you in making uterine and breast tissue. Also, protein helps you make blood (remember your blood volume increases 60% when you're pregnant), which is how your baby gets oxygen. You want to eat at least 70 grams of protein per day. You also need carbs—they are what give you energy. Whole grains are a great carb which contains fiber. This will help things to keep moving without plugging your bowels. Pregnancy constipation can be a problem and eating fiber is the fix.

F—Fats: Help your baby's development because they are your baby's main energy source for growth. Fats are essential for your baby's vitamin absorption (and yours, too). Good fats like DHA (an omega 3 fatty acid) help your baby with brain and eye development. You can find DHA in eggs and salmon.

Take Action

Grab a journal or piece of paper and a pen. A journal is a fantastic way to figure things out anytime in life but especially when you're pregnant.

So here are a couple questions for ya:

1. What hit you most from everything Dr. Hays' said? What surprised you, what are you thinking about? Start writing and just write for 3 minutes (with no interruptions), then come back to #2 below.

2. Is your provider someone who sits down with you and takes the time to get to know YOU as a woman? Or someone who points you to a packet of information when you have questions and hustles out the door after your 10 minute appointment because of their busy schedule? If you don't know, find out. If your instincts are telling you to break up with your provider, do it. Find someone else. It's as easy as googling OB/GYNs or midwives in your geographical area, asking *better questions* of your friends or friends' friends, reading reviews online and then setting appointments to interview them.

Take Action (continued)

*Better questions just mean more detailed questions, helping you get closer to the end result you want. Ask more detailed questions by asking open ended questions instead of closed ended questions.

For example: ask your friend open-ended questions like: "So how did Dr. _____ make you feel supported? What did they do? How did they ask you what you wanted? What didn't they do? Can you run me through what Dr. _____ was doing throughout your labor and birth—when they came in, how often, what they said, etc."

Closed-ended questions are ones with a yes or no answer. We call those "time wasters" 'cause you don't get answers that will help you make better decisions. Like "Did you like your doctor?" "Was your midwife good?"

Open-ended questions tell you a story. Date your doctor (or midwife) mamas!

Great work mama, now head on over to Lesson #2.

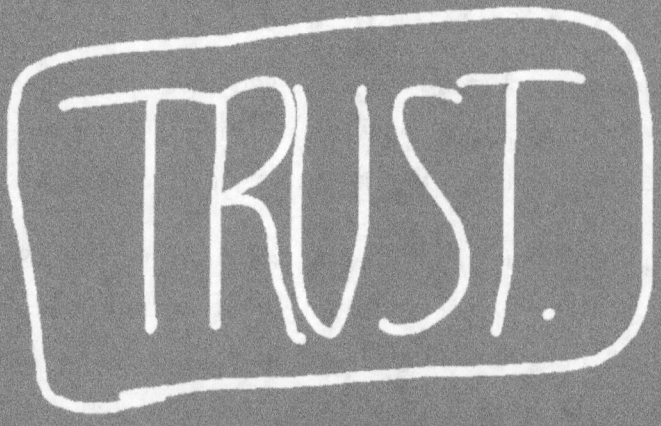

"Developing a relationship with your practitioner and a trust in your body are probably the two most important things that a woman can do when she's pregnant. Trust that your body knows what to do!"

Dr. Stuart Fischbein (dad of 4, top Ob/Gyn)

"How to be Fearless during Pregnancy & Birth"

-with Dr. Stuart Fischbein, top Ob/Gyn, dad of four

Sarah: We're learning about fear and how to be fearless in pregnancy and childbirth, and even after birth. Here with us is Dr. Fischbein. He's been an OB/GYN for 25 years. He's the co-founder of the Woman's Place, which is a really cool, innovative model of collaborative care with midwives and doctors, and he's the co-author of "Fearless Pregnancy: Wisdom and Reassurance from a Doctor, a Midwife, and a Mom."

He's also a dad of four kids, has a lot to teach us about pregnancy and birth, and is really passionate about the midwifery model of care. We're going to find out why an OB is so passionate about midwives, and why he thinks women have the right to know their options in pregnancy and childbirth.

From all your experience as a dad and an OB, what are you most inspired to share with expectant moms?

Dr. Fischbein: Pregnancy is not an illness.

We've had three generations of American women who have been sort of confused or — I hate to use the word brainwashed, but I'll use the word brainwashed — to believe that if it weren't for medical technology and hospital settings, that our species would have probably been extinct long ago.

And that women *need* to give birth in a hospital, that giving birth outside of the hospital is ridiculed, archaic, or stupid.

Those sorts of myths are played over and over again, and if you repeat these things enough times, you develop a culture that actually starts believing that those myths are based on evidence.

What is really true is that for women who have no problems with their pregnancy, the evidence does not suggest that at all. As a matter of fact, the evidence suggests that it's not safe necessarily or safer necessarily to give birth in a hospital. So the idea that pregnancy is an illness is something that myself, the midwives I work with, several other physicians in the community, and physicians nationwide are trying to "repackage" this message.

We're trying to brand the issues in such a way that people start to ask the proper questions to get the best answers. Like ... *"why are we being told if it wasn't for these interventions our baby might die? Or that I'm going to have a terrible outcome or some problem unless I have these interventions?"*

All these fear-based issues have become an art in the forefront. That would be the number one thing.

Sarah: That totally leads in to our topic, which is fear. If we're brought up believing that "the system" is what's really going to get us through pregnancy and birth, that we need to just roll over and endure it rather than find a way to thrive in it, then it seems like a no-brainer... of course we'll feel fear. So what can you share with women to diminish that fear?

Dr. Fischbein: That's a really a great question.

I'm going to start with sort of an example that we often use. Every week at the Sanctuary, we meet couples that are looking at options.

The Sanctuary Birth and Family Wellness Center is a collaborative practice between licensed midwives and doctors, myself, and then doctors who back us at hospitals, where we offer people a birthing center or home birthing.

One of the founders of the sanctuary often says this, *"First of all, birth is a very special time in a woman's life. She may do it two, three times, maybe once. It's extremely memorable. That baby is only going to be born once. It's a monumental experience for any woman that's gone through it, whether it's at home or in a hospital. It's life-changing, and we treat it as if it's having your appendix out. Birth needs to be thought of in a different way."*

One example she uses to compare and bring home this point are weddings — weddings and birth are probably the two most memorable moments in a woman's life. We have no trouble spending $20,000, $50,000, or even $100,000 on our wedding.

But when we're pregnant, we look at our insurance card. We take out our [insurance] book. We say I've got to deliver at this hospital and use this group of doctors, and I've got to do what they tell me, and I'm going to go here, and I'm going to have this blood test, and I'm going to have this, and I know I've got to have an IV, and I'm going to come in, and I can't eat anything, and that's just the way it's done.

And we accept that.

We have to step back. Maybe we need to change how we look at birth, and look at it as an *event* rather than as a medical problem.

Imagine there was such a thing as wedding insurance. From the time you were 18 years old, you paid $100 a month to an insurance company, and when the big wedding day finally came, your entire wedding was covered except for a small co-payment. Wouldn't that be great?

However, what if they've decided that you could only eat *this* kind of food, and you could only have it at *this* facility, and you couldn't pick out the dress you wanted, and you were to invite people you didn't like? Would any of us accept that?

The answer is no, of course we wouldn't. But that's exactly what we accept when it comes to the birth of our baby!

So maybe we need to rethink it. The first thing you have to understand is that normal birth is not an illness. Birth doesn't need to be feared.

There are things that can go wrong in pregnancy and hospitals and newborn intensive care units *certainly* have a place in modern medical obstetrics, but not for everybody.

People need to be given a choice. Some people given a choice will choose that anyway. But other people given a choice will choose not to go to the hospital, and if everybody knew what the evidence states and what the statistics are, then they can make a choice that suits them as an individual.

We end up sort of putting everybody into a package. Everybody is the same. It's one size fits all policies and protocols and procedures in hospitals. That's not the way you make birth memorable.

Sarah: Is it just unique to our American culture? Is there anywhere else in the world where this fear dominates birth?

Dr. Fischbein: It's different in other countries. In the European countries, it's different—they have a different model of obstetrical care. But anywhere you have media, anywhere you have competition for internet advertising, TV advertising, and 600 channels on your direct TV, they're going to want to draw your attention. And how do you draw someone's attention to something? You market something that's interesting.

Normal birth is less interesting than problems.

You don't ever see a headline in *The New York Times* that says "All Planes Landed Safely Today." Yet, most planes land safely, that's the norm. But when we have plane crashes, especially if you have video, then it's spectacular.

Then you see it over and over and over again. People who see this over and over and over again start to build up a fear. It's particularly pervasive in our culture also because—and I know that my friends in the American Legal System are not going to always like what I have to say, but we do have a litigious culture.

People are encouraged to sue. Sue for economic reasons, medical legal reasons, there are expediency reasons why we're all stuck in this rut, and maybe we'll go through those as the interview goes along. But yes, it is more pervasive in the United States culture than it is in most of the Western European countries.

Sarah: Is it possible as a woman who is pregnant to over prepare for pregnancy and kind of induce stress or fear by just being too prepared or knowing too much about everything that could happen?

Dr. Fischbein: Well, that answer is a yes, but also, a well-educated patient is better off than somebody who's ignorant. You're far more likely to have irrational fear if you are not educated. But yes, if you read too much. And there are many sources of both in the internet and the books that are fear-based. The most pervasive or the most well-read book in pregnancy, which I won't mention, which everyone gets at least one copy of when they get pregnant, is a fear-based book. It makes you worry. It makes you more concerned. But I would never say that educating yourself is a bad thing.

Sarah: So using a filter as you're taking in information is probably a good idea.

Dr. Fischbein: How to find the filter is a more difficult thing.

Developing a relationship with your practitioner, a trust in your body, are probably the two most important things that a woman can do when she's pregnant. Trust that your body knows what to do.

Your body has been biologically developing over a million years. It knows how to reproduce. It knows how to deliver a baby, and if you let it do that, then it will do it right most of the time.

If you have a practitioner that you trust, whether it be a doctor, a midwife, family practitioner, your grandmother... if you have that trust and you have that confidence, then fear has a tougher time getting in.

One of the ways to determine whether you have a good relationship with your practitioner is to feel like you can ask questions without feeling like you're getting the eye roll, or the short answer, or the *"don't-worry-about-that,"* or a patronizing comment.

No question is stupid in pregnancy.

If you're made to feel as if your questions are stupid, it's maybe time to look elsewhere for another practitioner. If you feel uncomfortable just asking a question in that setting, you're going to feel less empowered by the time you're in labor.

And it really is about the empowerment of the woman in her own body, in her own sort of primitive limbic brain, to trust that her own body will work. If you start to think too much, your higher brain functions take over with their reflexive processes and inner fear.

This is sort of a weak analogy, but stress can cause an upset stomach, right?

It's not that you ate anything different, it's that your body puts out hormones that change how your body responds. Your body's interfering with the normal process of digestion, which is something that you don't have to think about.

Labor is also something you shouldn't have to think about. The minute you start thinking, you interfere with labor.

Sarah: That leads to my next question. Can you give us examples from all your experience how fear has held women back while they're in labor?

Dr. Fischbein: Sure. I would liken it with the example of other mammals. We give birth to our children live born, from the uterus, through the vagina and into the world.

If you look at other mammals and how they give birth, they go off to some quiet place. They don't go to the center of the freeway. They certainly don't go to "the emergency room." They go off to some quiet place, and who do they go with? Nobody. They go off alone.

As a matter of fact, the other members of the herd tend to leave them alone. They tend to not want to be interrupted, and if they want to walk around, they walk around. They're not confined in any one space.

As a matter of fact, it's really rare for a laboring mammal to just sit down until they're ready to give birth. If they're hungry, they eat.

And if the predator comes nearby, if they're disturbed, then their higher brain takes over. They put out adrenaline. Adrenaline stops the secretion of oxytocin, which is your own natural hormone causing your uterus to contract.

Contractions space out, the animal gets up, does its fight-or-flight response or runs away. And after the thing that's caused them to be stressed or fearful is gone, they settle back down, find their place, and give birth. We, as a species, do it all wrong.

Everything we do in the hospital birthing world is sort of counterintuitive to what nature designed. We leave our nest to get in our car and drive to an emergency room to get put in a wheelchair and taken upstairs to labor and delivery, where we're asked to sign a bunch of consent forms. Not very primitive brain stuff. We're asked to pee in a cup before changing into a hospital gown. We're not wearing our own jammies or we're not walking around naked like we might do in our own home.

We're put into bed. We're strapped in bed with these monitors on our belly so they can watch the baby. Often, we'll put an IV in your arm then put the blood pressure cuff on your arm. You're not allowed to eat. If you have to go to the bathroom, you ask permission. You're being interrupted constantly for vital signs and being asked questions.

You have people sitting around the room. Your husband, your mother-in-law, your grandmother are sitting in chairs staring at you. Actually, they're not really staring at you, they're staring at the machine next to you. You're all looking at it.

This is so counter with what nature designed. *It's a setup that triggers the stress and fear-based hormones that'll interrupt your labor.* It's no wonder we have such a high rate of Pitocin usage (Pitocin is the drug that induces labor) and then epidural usage.

Pitocin is painful. It causes the contractions to be a little stronger, a little more close together. Part of the reason it's painful is because you're not allowed to get up. You're not allowed to walk around. You're not allowed to get in the shower or use other methods of pain control, so you end up asking for an epidural, and now you can't move at all.

You can't feel your legs. Your blood pressure drops. Your baby doesn't like that. They have to turn off the Pitocin. Then they turn the Pitocin back on. The baby's heart rate goes down again and they rush you down the hall for a c-section, and thank God we have the operating room there. Isn't that great!

And it was all sort of iatrogenically (that word means- caused by physicians) caused by the whole process of interrupting that primitive response your body will do on its own. Just like other mammals.

If you can avoid the fear, avoid it. Fear interrupts that whole labor process, which then leads to all these interventions (this is what some people call the "cascade of interventions"), which results in our high rates of medicalized birth—forceps, vacuums, c-sections, and a sort of a lack of satisfaction of your birth process.

When you sit back weeks later and you start to analyze what happened, you have a lot of questions. They're unanswered. Questions like… *"Did I really need that? Did I really—was this really the way it was supposed to be?"*

And when we have a c-section rate approaching 35% in this country, to believe that one-third of women are not capable of doing what nature designed is astonishing. There should be more people challenging it, and I think that with programs like this and other avenues of getting the word out, then people are beginning to start to wake up. I mean home birth in this country is still less than 1% of birth, but it's picking up.

And high-profile people like Ricki Lake and others give people the idea to stop and think for a second and ask questions like *"maybe there's a better way..."*

Sarah: Dr. Fischbein, is it possible for a woman to have a hospital birth in a way that isn't stress and adrenaline filled and to have a soothing natural wonderful experience? Have you seen that and who are those women who have that?

Dr. Fischbein: Yes, it's possible. It's not easy because hospitals have policies and have timetables. They interfere with that primitive stuff that we were talking about. The women that do that are again the women that I said earlier are comfortable in their own skin. They're confident in their body's ability to labor and give birth. They have a good support system.

They have a trusting practitioner who's onboard with them. They very likely have a doula. I can't stress enough for people that give birth in a hospital, but you're far less likely to have interventions or need a cesarean section when you hire a doula.

So anybody who chooses to give birth there, whether it's for medical reasons or just because you feel safer there, hire a doula.

And you can design—and you can come in with a birth plan, and you may get a nurse that's great. And remember, your primary care giver at a hospital is not your doctor, all right.

Your doctor is at home or in the office, and the nurse is your primary care giver. Nurses do change shifts, but if you get lucky and you get a really good nurse, you can have a great experience.

Sometimes it's a crapshoot because nurses come in all shapes and sizes. They have good days and they have bad days, so you don't know which you're going to get. That's why if you have a doula, she can act as an intermediary to prevent you from being drawn out of your primitive space.

But yes, it can be done...

And then you can ask for delayed cord clamping.

*Note: we delve more into delayed cord clamping in our next book, "Birth Book #2."

You can ask for no separation of the baby, because there's no reason after a baby is born, that in the first hour, the baby needs to be separated from its mom.

Again, going back to our nature model, when a baby horse is born, do they come and take it away from the mother? Do they come with tooth clamps and cut the cord? No. I mean I've seen baby horses walking around while dragging their placenta along the ground. They fall off eventually.

That's not a problem. The baby and the mother never separate. The mother licks the baby, smells the baby, bonds with the baby, and the baby is bonding just the same with its mom. As soon as the baby can stand up, it goes for the nipple. That's what should be done.

There's no reason that you have to weigh a baby, dry the baby off, put a little hat on the baby, clamp the cord and cut the cord. Those things are done in the hospitals partly because they have time tables. The hospital staff has to move on. They have to do their charting. There's so much charting in the hospitals, because of the legal stuff that goes on.

And part of it is done because of a saying by Thomas Paine from the American Revolution... *"The long habit of not thinking something is wrong gives the superficial appearance of it being right."*

And if the habit was always to take the baby from the mother, and dry the baby off, swaddle the baby, and then hand the baby back to the mother...that's the way it's done.

No one thinks, *"Why are we doing that? Why are we even taking the baby away from the mother in the first place?"*

Nature didn't design the baby to have to be taken away from the mother except in those rare cases where babies aren't doing well, and resuscitation or something by an ICU team is important. Fine. But on rare cases, even when babies are mildly suppressed, the best resuscitation that could happen for a baby is to stay connected to the placenta of the mother. While the baby's outside and trying to learn how to breathe, and taking its first breath, and looking around, it's still getting oxygen and nutrients in volume from the mother (*volume is blood from the mom's placenta).

As a matter of fact, when babies are born, a certain percentage of their blood volume has actually been squeezed into the placenta, and if you cut the cord immediately after the birth, you're actually depriving the baby of something that belongs to the baby.

So yes, it can happen, but it only happens to well-educated people. Otherwise, the system kicks in and takes over.

Sarah: So let's compare for a moment the patients you've had who were fearless, who were educated, who were prepared, who trusted their bodies, and who were active participants in their own birth process to the women you've seen who just kind of gave themselves over to the system. What differences do you see in these women as far as how they feel and how they perceive themselves in general?

Dr. Fischbein: I think it has a fairly obvious answer. To some women, birth is just an event that goes on, and it's not that important. They deal with their lives differently, and again, every woman is an individual.

But if I had to generalize, women that have empowering births... feel great going into birth. They have a more loving relationship with their child. They have more connection with their baby. They have a more loving relationship with their spouse or their partner. They feel stronger. They feel there's no question about their birth. They don't look back and say, geez, I wonder if I could have done this differently. There's no sort of regret. I can't tell you how many times in interviews that we do or when I see a new client, and they come in, and they start to tell me about their birth story.

First of all, halfway through their story, I could finish the story for them. I've heard the same thing so many times.

But there's such a question in their mind and they don't feel like some of the things that happened to them were necessary.

And they have a regret about that.

Sometimes they even have anger, anger at themselves for not moving forward, anger at their practitioner, even anger at their spouse, or sometimes their spouse has a feeling of helplessness watching his beloved wife sort of be forced into this tract, and today, at a meeting, one of the husbands said, *"You know, if we're in a labor room and the doctor says we need a c-section, who am I to argue with the doctor?"*

Again, getting back to the trusting relationship thing.

So there's a real helplessness, a real feeling of guilt sometimes, anger sometimes, and frustration that you see in women who don't go through the process of empowerment.

A perfect example is when a woman transfers from a home birth after everything we've tried at home doesn't work and she goes to the hospital. If she ends up at the hospital having a cesarean section after whatever they do at the hospital doesn't work, the chance of her having a satisfying experience is so much greater because she knows that the cesarean section was necessary. The baby's path brought them to the cesarean section and every option was taken, as opposed to the woman who is three days overdue and induced by her doctor, for being three days overdue or the *"I-think-your-baby's-getting-big-syndrome."* This happens all the time. She ends up with the Pitocin epidural cascade of intervention we talked about earlier, resulting in a cesarean section. She's left wondering what would have happened if I would have just waited three or four more days? And they always wonder.

Sarah: Why is an OB so passionate about the midwifery style of care? Why are you such a big proponent of this?

Dr. Fischbein: I have to tell you that when I finished my residency program in the early '80s, I had to no concept of any other way to do it than the medical model by which I was trained. I was the gung-ho resident.

I was the administrative chief resident at Cedars Sinai. I came into practice and I thought I knew everything. I'll tell you, my evolution was a slow process. If you would have asked me 25 years ago if I would have been sitting here today with you having this conversation, I would have thought you were out of your mind.

I looked at people who wanted to have a home birth, who wanted to bury their placenta or make their placenta into capsules, or do these sorts of things as loony tunes. I really thought these people were out of their mind.

But as fortune would have it, when I started my practice, I was approached by some midwives and asked to be their backup physician, and of course, I'm building a practice from the ground up.

I'm not going to turn away the potential, you know, seeing new patients and developing new relationships. I said, *"Sure."*

And over time, you know, over the next ten years, I realized that everything that I learned—not everything—but most of the things that I learned for low-risk pregnancies or normal pregnancies, I had to unlearn because quite frankly, I had no training in normal pregnancy.

But the definition of an obstetrician is somebody who's trained in surgical birth, in surgery. I never had a lecture in eight years of medical student residency on nutrition.

And not one lecture on breastfeeding. I wasn't prepared to deal with preventative healthcare. I was trained in fixing problems.

Then I saw that normal birth doesn't require a whole lot of interventions. I would be backing three or four women a month for a certain midwife, and it would go six months before I had a transport and think *"Where are all these women? What happened to them? Did they go someplace else?"*

No, they all delivered at home. They all did great. So after ten years of doing this, this is when I founded the Woman's Place because I saw that the collaboration between midwives and physicians was the best way to go. Midwives are trained in low-risk birth. Doctors don't even want to deal with that.

I mean we deal with it because financially, we need the money, and some of us actually love OB. I shouldn't say that they don't want to deal with it, but ultimately, we're not—our model isn't like that.

Our model allows about six to ten minutes for prenatal visits. Midwives allow an hour. It's a whole different model.

I saw that collaboration with midwives taking care of low-risk people, and then if something went wrong or somebody needed genetic screening, or somebody needed an ultrasound, or somebody is having twins, or baby ended up being breech, that was outside their scope of practice and that's exactly what I wanted to do. I found that fantastic.

It was an evolution. It wasn't just an epiphany one night. It was an evolution of the process of seeing it work. And also, I battled for common sense and evidence-based things to go on in hospitals, and I was rebuked over and over again. So I sort of developed a chip on my shoulder about *"why can't we do VBACs?"* It's evidence-based. It's supported by the American College of OB/GYN. It's supported by the National Institute of Health. Why can't I do breech deliveries?

I'm credentialed to do them. I know how to do them. Hospitals banned them. My midwives were banned for a year from the local hospital in Camarillo.

For safety reasons, was their answer.

The canard of safety. The welfare of humanity is always the alibi of tyrants, and they were saying that it was unsafe for midwives whose patients are all low risk to give birth, while OB/GYNs could still do these births at this hospital.

It was ludicrous. I realized at a point that I could bang my head against the wall and come up empty every time because I'm never going to win, or I could go off and I could try to start my own paradigm, which is commonsensical and give women an alternative. There's so much support for what we're doing, I feel good about my life now.

I feel good about my job. I'm happy to go to work. I'm happy to go to a birth. I never felt that way when I was driving into the parking lot at the hospital I was working at.

So if we try to tell women who are pregnant to live a good life, to be stress free, to eat well, to sleep well, to have good relationships with their partners, we have to walk the talk.

And I wasn't. And I think most obstetricians are not walking the talk. The burnout rate's pretty high. When they get a phone call at 2 in the morning and someone's in labor, it's *"oh crap!"* It's not..."*how wonderful.*"

And that's the difference, and that's sort of how I ended up where I am right now, and I love speaking about it. You know what? It makes me feel good to have people come up to me and tell me that I'm doing something good.

As an obstetrician, you get a few accolades, but really, all you hear about are the cases that go wrong, the people angry, people who don't want to pay their bill, that sort of thing. That's the stuff that you get e-mails about or you get certified letters about. I don't want to get certified letters about those things. Doctors hate certified letters. We have certified letter cold sweats.

Sarah: You've been an OB for 25 years. I'm sure you have a lot of amazing birth stories. Can you share with us one or two birth stories that really taught you something about birth?

Dr. Fischbein: Yes, I can. As a matter of fact, I can think of somebody very unique. Her name is Becky, and she is sort of in the fringe of the birth community. And she's had three previous births. The first birth was a cesarean section, and then her second and third births were vaginal birth after cesarean section, both at home. In her fourth pregnancy, it turned out that she had twins, right.

So she couldn't find anyone to do her twins VBAC in a hospital. I was willing to do them in the home setting, and I've done several other twins in the home setting. She was unique because at the time that she got to her term, both her babies were in the breech presentation.

Breech-breech twins. Nobody does breech-breech twins. Nobody does breech-vertex twins. Very few people do vertex-breech twins unless they're head first-head first, which you call vertex-vertex. A lot of people are just going straight to c-section for twins, but the evidence doesn't support that.

And so we did a literature search, and we looked around, and we found that there is no evidence against doing breech-breech twins, that as a matter of fact, there are some anecdotal reports before and stuff that say that in the woman who meets a certain criteria who's well educated, who chooses that path, and a practitioner was willing to support her, you can do that.

But no one would allow her to have that done in the hospital, so where was she going to do that? The only place she could do it if she's going to do it is at home. She trusted her body and she trusted our team, and she had a beautiful birth.

Her baby was born on February 14th a little after 10 p.m. in the evening. The next baby was born—and that was in the water in the tub. The next baby was born shortly after midnight on February 15th in her bedroom, and everything went beautifully.

Could something have gone wrong? Sure. But generally, when you trust labor and you follow things, and you don't push beyond limits, things don't go wrong.

So that for me was a wonderful thing, and we were able to give her the option, and since that time, we've done lots of breeches, because breeches in the Southern California area don't have any option other than this wonderful old doctor at Glendale who does hospital breeches, but otherwise, breeches are automatically c-section. But breech is just a variation of normal.

There are countless births where you see the woman grab her own baby, pull it up on her chest and hold it there. You see the look about her face, the tears in her eyes, the look on her partner's face.

My favorite time in a birth when I used to attend birth in the hospital was when everything was sort of done, was sitting in the chair in the corner of the room, filling out the chart, and just quietly looking at the couple with their new baby and maybe their other children would come into the room by then, and just in seeing that this is a family bonding event, it is.

It doesn't have to be the same as taking out your appendix, and when we do a c-section, and we separate the mother from the baby, and the baby goes to the nursery, and the father is separated from the family, and everyone else is in the waiting room. You're looking at the baby through the glass. This is not what nature designed. This is not what was intended. It should be avoided as much as possible. It should not be nurtured.

As I said earlier, there's always a chance. When this is necessary, it's important, but it should not be the law.

Sarah: I really appreciate your time, Dr. Fischbein, and your passion for women, babies, and this whole experience of empowering women to know that they do have choices and to really get the whole scoop on what their choices and options are.

Don't let those fears fester, acknowledge them and get them out...doing that will depower them and give YOU the upper hand!

Supporting Evidence

Your environment affects <u>everything</u> you do. It affects your performance at work, school, home, sports, vacation...and most definitely birth! It's that mind-body connection. Your brain sees even the smallest of things and triggers your body to respond.

Think how many gazillions of dollars casinos have spent on improving the "casino environment" for their gamblers (brighter lighting, carpet colors, likeable sounds, appealing textures and sights, feel good smells...on and on). Casinos know if their environment helps people *feel* a certain way, people will respond by staying and gambling more. *Even with the pain of losing money.*

Or maybe a better analogy is a spa. The low lights, the scents of lavender and eucalyptus, soothing music and those fluffy bath robes. Ahh, it just makes you take a few deep breaths and relax.

It's the same sitch with birth. The mind-body connection is real, your mind is affecting your body right now—it's just basic human physiology. The mind-body connection is in full effect and it totally makes all the sense in the world, doesn't it? Our body follows our mind!

There is evidence from the US Cochrane Center at the Johns Hopkins School of Public Health showing how hospitals' "institutional settings" can affect birth. This study[iv] looked at 11,795 women and concluded... *"When compared to conventional institutional settings, alternative settings were associated with reduced likelihood of medical interventions, increased likelihood of spontaneous vaginal birth, increased maternal satisfaction, and greater likelihood of continued breastfeeding at one to two months postpartum, with no apparent risks to mother or baby."*

This is not a dig on hospitals. It's to make you aware that all birth settings, especially hospitals, are not created equal (birth centers, too).

This is info to find out early on. If you know you'll feel safer in a hospital, some hospitals have received a "mother-friendly" designation (ask to find out if any near you have). To receive this designation, 10 steps have to be met- (you can see the entire list of steps about half-way down the page at the Coalition For Improving

Maternity Services.) For example, they hide machines that aren't being used, they don't hook you up to machines that beep or force you to lie down unless absolutely medically required, and they encourage you to bring in "comforts" from home (music, food, pictures, essential oils like lavender or jasmine, clothes that you feel most comfortable in, etc.). *They do a great job helping you feel like you're not in a hospital.* Other hospitals make zero effort.

The point is your surroundings have a huge effect on how you feel and your level of fear. Fear affects your mind, which controls your body (less pain, faster labor, etc.), which determines what happens during birth. We explain how your brain triggers your body's fight-or-flight response on our website yourbabybooty.com.[v]

Dr. Fischbein also talked about how important it is to have a doula for you to get *the best maternity care through labor and birth*. We really went into detail about all the super meaningful benefits of doulas (28% decreased chance of c-section, 31% lower chance of needing to be induced with Pitocin, 34% more likely to feel good about your whole birth experience, less likely to need pain medication, less likely to have to send your baby to special needs nursery, etc.) in lesson one with Dr. Hays. If you haven't already, read that lesson and the evidence for using a doula (review of 22 trials including over 15,000 women). [vi]

In Short

Before I was even married, I would think about having a family one day. I would always think that having a baby must be so incredibly painful and that I was a wimp. I questioned if I really even wanted to endure the pain of giving birth. But then I would say to myself, *"but people have been doing this for a gazillion years...over and over again. It must not be that bad."*

I know that so many women look at birth kinda like Mount Everest. They stand in the city of Katmandu and look up at the mountain and think, *"how am I ever going to get to the top?"* It may be daunting but it's do-able. Everything is do-able if you have a strong enough *why*. Step number one is to banish the fear. One contraction at a time takes you to the top. One foot in front of the other.

Dr. Fischbein mentions that birth is not like having your appendix out. It's not a problem. It's an event—a life altering one for the better. Becoming a parent will expose you to joy that you never knew was possible. It will also test you like there's no tomorrow (just ask anyone with a two-year-old). I came to realize when I did become pregnant for the first time, that to take control of fear, I had to filter out the negative.

It's very challenging when we're bombarded by social media, by TV media, by print media 24/7. But I found that turning things off, and even asking people not to share their scary, crazy birth story, helped my frame of mind. Instead, I would feed myself positive fuel. Just as the climbers who summit Mt. Everest have to feed themselves the best nutrients to fuel their bodies to the max, I did the same. Learning how my body was made to birth my baby was my positive fuel. It's a huge confidence booster to learn precisely *how* a woman's body is uniquely built to do this—to birth babies.

Take Action

1. What stood out to you most from everything Dr. Fischbein shared? The first thing you think about right now, whatever it is, just go...write for at least 3 minutes. Give yourself the freedom to get out whatever is buried in your head. Then come back to #2 below...

2. Learn how your body is uniquely designed to do this life-giving job. Spend 1 hour a week focusing on how your body & baby work together. Start reading our next book, Birth Book #2. It's incredible info that will completely change how you feel about your body!

    You'll be blown away with everything your body does, will do, and is capable of doing. It all adds up to serious confidence during labor and birth. You'll be one fearless birthing mama in a world that thrives on drama and fear. That's huge.

3. Share your worries and concerns with your spouse or bestie. One doctor told me, "It all comes out during labor." It's true. Whatever could hold you back, you want to write it down to confront it now. Fears and worries (no matter how silly or how big they might be) can literally roadblock your labor[vii]. And make it come to a screeching halt.

Take Action (continued)

Thankfully, it's avoidable! By getting it out, you depower it. You expose it. Your fears are untruths about the future played over and over 'til they own you.

Okay, so draw 2 columns on a page in your journal. On one side write down what you're most fearful of. Now on the other side what you're most excited about. Talk about each one of those fears with your spouse (or bestie, midwife, or doula—after all, they've seen it all!) in the next 3 days. This 10-minute exercise helps you avoid having fear driving you down a road you don't want to be on. I know this can be tough, but you'll be so glad you did it!

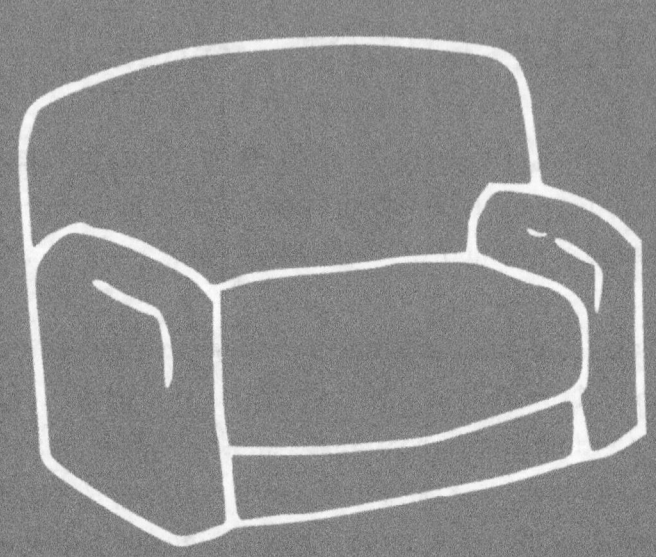

"...this was a doctor who was comfortable with the idea that I had done a lot of research and I wasn't a moron..."

Kate Glynn, mama of 2

lesson three

"OB/GYN or Midwife? How To Choose the Best Doctor or Midwife For You"

- Kate Glynn, mom of two

Sarah Blight: Are you sure you're with the best Doctor or Midwife? Or maybe you're just starting to check into it. How do you know you're with the right Midwife or Doctor?

Kate Glynn is here to teach you how to avoid her bad experience with doctor #1 and how to have her a-m-a-z-i-n-g experience with doctor #2. She's the mom of two kids. So, Kate, why is it so important that we carefully choose the right doctor or midwife and how do we actually do it?

Kate Glynn: There are literally few things more intimate than having a baby, right? This is a person who you're going to see at least once a month for the next year of your life. This Is the person who you need to trust completely, and I think also because in childbirth, it's so important to advocate for yourself, that I think having someone that can hear you and is willing to listen, is super, super important.

Sarah: Why was it important for you to choose the right person?

Kate: So, my personal experience was actually with my first kiddo. My insurance provider said, *"Okay, here's a doctor"* and I took that name and I went and—I actually, immediately had that little voice in my head going, *"This is not the right person"* and I didn't listen. Primarily because I didn't want to go through the hassle of talking to the insurance people, changing doctors, blah, blah, blah—and I kind of dragged my feet and before I knew it, we had done the twenty-week ultrasound, and at that point it just seemed like too much, too late...

And I thought..."*I'm just sticking with her.*"

But—it's something that I regret to this day. Specifically what happened, we confirmed the pregnancy at about 6 weeks, and at 6 weeks she said, *"Okay, so we're going to induce you at 38 weeks."*

I said, *"Why?"*

And she goes, *"Oh, well, it's better that way"* and I said, *"Okay, why? Is there something wrong with the shape of my pelvis, am I going to have a really big kid? What are you not telling me?"*

She says, *"No, no, no! Everything's fine. It's just better that way."*

And I said, *"Noooo, you're not inducing me, I'm going to go full term. Whenever the baby's ready, the baby's going to come out."* And we went back and forth and back and forth and she was just sort of like, *"It will be fine, it will be fine,"* and it seemed like she was very used to patients who wouldn't think and just say ... "Oh yes, Doctor! Whatever you say, Doctor!" And I was not that patient, so there was instantly this sort of bad vibe.

I was convinced I got my point through and said, *"If I go past 41 weeks, then we can start talking about induction, but never before that."* Then at my 37 week appointment, I went in and she said, *"Okay, so I scheduled an induction for you next Wednesday. So check yourself into the hospital on Tuesday night,"* and I said, *"Whoa! Whoa! Whoa! Whoa! Whoa! No, no, no!"* and so we went around and around again.

My son ended up being five days late, and in the meantime at 33 weeks, she put me on, what do they call it, it's like modified bed rest, because I was 80% effaced and 30% dilated at 33 weeks. And so she said, *"You know, premature labor, bed rest,"* and as a first-time mom, I was thinking, *"Oh god! I don't wanna have a preemie."*

Then my son was five days late. He was perfectly healthy and I ended up having an emergency c-section because he had the cord wrapped around his neck three times.

My doctor was not there, it was the attending doctor on call who ended up delivering. My son was born on a Saturday, and when I saw her again on Monday morning during her rounds, she said... *"I told you, you should have induced at 38 weeks. If you had listened to me, this wouldn't have happened."*

And I remember thinking, *"If I didn't have 15 staples in my abdomen right now, I'd be coming across the bed at you!"*

How dare you! You know?

Sarah: So even as a first time mom, having never gone through it before, you knew what you wanted. Why didn't you want to be induced at 38 weeks? Why was that important to you?

Kate: So—I guess my fundamental belief is that—I think, you know, modern medicine has been fantastic, and obviously there are a lot of pregnancies that wouldn't make it without intervention, but if everything is going normally, as I kind of knew it was, then I really believe in minimal intervention. Does that make sense?

It's in a strange way the same reason I buy organic food. Why fix it if it's not broken?

I really have faith in my body and faith in women's bodies, in general, and certainly there are situations in which medical intervention is absolutely necessary, and I think, you know, the c-section was absolutely necessary. I don't think my son would have survived without it.

With that said, I think there's this huge culture right now of making women afraid of childbirth and afraid of pregnancy and treating it almost like a disease, and I think that just takes away from the whole experience and I just really think that's a negative.

Sarah: Let's go to baby number two, because you have two kids. What did you learn from experience one that you said to yourself, okay, I'm not doing that again?

Kate: I was much more careful about selecting a doctor. When I got pregnant with Fiona, with number two, I was in Corpus Christi, Texas.

There was very, very little choice. There were no birthing centers, there was one practicing midwife, but no physician back up. She only did home births with no physician back-up, so I just felt like my options were restricted. But having my first son, I met a lactation consultant/doula, and so I really used her. When I got pregnant with number two, I called her and said, *"Okay, I want a doctor who's going to let me VBAC"*, which was hard to find anyway...

Sarah: Which means vaginal birth after Cesarean section, for those of you who don't know.

Kate: I wanted a doctor who was going to support my no meds, minimal intervention stance and I knew that was going to be hard to come by. So I really leaned on her to find somebody. I got very lucky.

She introduced me to this wonderful female doctor who had children around the same age. She was fantastic, but during the first visit she said, *"I'm sorry, I can't deliver your baby."* I was like, *"Oh."* And it was because she was pregnant, too, and was due eight weeks before I was.

So, fair enough, she recommended her partner in her practice, who was also her personal OB, who was a guy, which I wasn't used to at all! I always thought I'd have a female OB, but his name was Dr. Wilder, and he, as far as I'm concerned, is the best thing since sliced bread!

Great doctor! I was so comfortable talking to him about what was important to me and not only was I able to advocate for myself, but I knew that if I said something, he was also going to advocate for me. Does that make sense?

He was on my side, he was the one telling the hospital, *"Yes, she can disconnect from the monitors and walk around, because that's what she wants,"* you know? He was such an amazing ally, it was a completely different experience.

Sarah: Did you feel like he was different just from the fact that he didn't really assert himself into your care?

Kate: And I think that's exactly it. He was much more willing, almost like a therapist, to step back and let me talk and then mold the experience to what I needed it to be. And my first OB, with my son, was very much like *"This is how I do it and you shall do it my way or otherwise,"* kind of thing. So a very, very different vibe.

Sarah: So that experience, how did that translate into your childbirth experience? What did that feel like?

Kate: So empowering. I mean, it was really, really good. He was very calming—for example, I've heard this statistic that if you're VBACing, you're twice as likely to experience uterine rupture, right? So I said, *"Okay, so I really want to VBAC, but is this true?"* He said, *"Yes, it's true! It goes up from 0.4 to 0.8%."*

He was very matter of fact. He was the guy who told me, if you're going to give up either caffeine or alcohol during pregnancy, give up caffeine, because a glass of wine once a week isn't going to hurt the baby. But if you get into a cycle of needing caffeine now, then when you're breastfeeding a newborn you're sure as heck going to need it. The baby's going to get it through your breast milk, and the baby's never going to sleep. So if you're going to go either route, cut out caffeine.

So, he seemed to be this very common sense, very chill guy.

Sarah: You seem like a confident, no-nonsense, let's cut straight to the point kind of person, so it seems like that would really work well for you?

Kate: It was really good. And I think my absolute favorite thing about him, which was also a complete contrast from my first experience, this was a doctor who was comfortable with the idea that I had done a lot of research and I wasn't a moron, you know?

Despite the fact that I'm not an MD, if I asked questions with a scientific slant to it, you know, he wasn't like, *"Oh, you silly little girl."* He would actually engage with me seriously and he wouldn't water down answers. He would actually talk in medical terms, assuming I would understand it. And if I didn't, I would ask a question. Not being patronized was really nice.

Sarah: So it seems like he treated you like a partner in this whole process?

Kate: Yep, that's exactly the way that I describe it!

Sarah: Like you're working together, you're both wanting the same things, which definitely would seem a lot more gratifying to anybody in any kind of an experience, whether you're birthing a baby or getting your car fixed? I mean, you just want to know

what's going on and have a normal conversation about why suggestions are being made, what the implications are of those suggestions, what the risks are, what the benefits are and what other options you might have. Just like in everything else we do, it seems like that would be a good thing.

So you said you realized you had chosen the wrong doctor from day one with your first child. What can women do if they're in your shoes right now and what advice would you give them if they're thinking, "*I know that feeling, this isn't the right provider for me*"?

Kate: I would say trust your instincts, and that's really what I didn't do. I had this little "instinctual ick" feeling and I didn't do anything with it, I didn't follow it. I regret that. So, I think, trust your instincts, and also before you go to that first OB appointment, do some research, you know?

It turns out when I was choosing my second OB, there were actually a lot of doctors who were willing to be interviewed before I selected them. And I think I interviewed four before I stumbled on this fantastic pair.

And the doctors who were not willing to be interviewed, I thought, "*Well, that's a sign,*" you know? So I think, definitely educate yourself. Know what you want.

I mean, if you're a person who wants a doctor who's going to be like, "*Okay, let's do pain management, let's do medication,*" you know? Then that's fine. Find the doctor that's going to fit you.

And if you're like me, and you want the opposite of that, do some research, talk to the doulas, talk to the lactation consultants, you know? Go talk to the La Leche League. All the crunchy, granola people you can find, and they're going to have the local "ins" to who the best people are to help you with what you want.

Sarah: That's a great tip. I do want to mention the fact that you were active military duty at this point. So if you're in the military system of healthcare and really feeling like you're hemmed in with your choices, then you're really not. You still have options. So how will a woman know if she is with THE right doctor or midwife for them?

Kate: For me it was two-fold. My pregnancy with my daughter was actually a more complicated pregnancy for me. Thank goodness everything turned out fine, but there were more issues during the pregnancy. And with everything that was going on, I just—I trusted him. It was very comfortable—I didn't think he was going to pull the wool over my eyes.

I knew if there was something really catastrophically wrong, he was going to tell me. So I had this incredible confidence in his integrity, you know? Just like you said earlier...I was a partner and he wasn't going to try to coddle me. The other thing, which was just amazing, was actually looking forward to seeing him every month!

And because of the complications, I actually got to see him every week for 21 weeks. So I actually looked forward to it, and I almost considered having a third, just so I could be his patient again—I miss Doctor Wilder!

Sarah: Now that is really saying something.

Kate: Yeah, it was amazing.

Sarah: So when you were interviewing those other three candidates, what was it that made you cross them off your list? Was it just another instinctual feeling or were there red flags?

Kate: One was an instinctual feeling. One of them was very simple. She just said she couldn't really take a new patient at this point, so she was going to have to fob me off on a partner.

So that was an easy one. One was that instinctual ick, and then if I remember correctly, the third one, I was very tempted, she was a new mom herself and actually had a pack-and-play in her personal office, and I thought, *"Okay, this is a person who—we're in the same place."* We just didn't quite click.

Sarah: There was no chemistry there?

Kate: Yeah. The chemistry was lacking. And I guess that I really lucked out in Doctor Wilder, because he was not the person I (originally) hired. It was his partner, who was also fantastic.

And I think it was easy for me to make the transition because I really loved my original doctor—her name was Dr. Canterbury, and I loved Dr. Canterbury for all the same reasons. So when she recommended Dr. Wilder, it was easy, it was like… *"Okay, I trust you."*

Sarah: Right, right, right, because she trusts her own baby and birth experience to this person, too.

Kate: Exactly.

Sarah: That's a huge vote of confidence, right there.

Kate: Absolutely, absolutely...

Sarah: Kate, thank you for sharing your experience with us, 'cause it's real, it's authentic, and it's really helpful!

In Short

Today I saw a man breaking into the vacant (for sale) house next door. So I got out of my car and tazed him. No, I didn't really do that...but I did ask him what the heck was going on. He said he was my new neighbor. I went inside and decided to call the cops because I just felt that something was off.

It turns out that I was wrong.

I called the cops on my new neighbors. Oopsadaisy. But what if I was right?

How often do we feel something in our guts and not follow through, not take action and look back with regret?

That was Kate, she knew from the first moment that she should switch providers and didn't listen to her gut Instinct.

What do your gut instincts tell you? Do you listen? Are you honed in on what you think or feel and then take action?

Kate's story resonates so much with me, partly because our stories share some similarities and partly because I hear from many, many, many women who look back on their births with regret. And that regret comes with a big tug in their heart that says *"Damn. I didn't know I could have had better or had different options... I knew something wasn't quite right. I wish I would have researched more."*

Most women don't know they can interview prospective doctors or midwives. YES. YES. YES, you can. And you should! ***Is there a more important job than helping you bring your baby into this crazy world? If there was ever a time for a job interview...it's now.***

Here are 5 questions to get you started as you interview providers:

1. How do you see your role as a doctor/midwife during my prenatal care and at my baby's birth?
2. How will we spend our time at appointments, beyond necessary physical care? (Will there be time to ask questions? Address concerns I have about my baby or myself? Talk about emotional issues? Nutrition? Other topics?)
3. How many of your patients end up with c-sections?
4. Why did you become a doctor/midwife?
5. What is the most important thing for me to know as I prepare to give birth?

Take Action

1. Take 3 minutes & write. What do you love about your provider, practice and/or hospital where you'll deliver (if applicable)? What aren't you thrilled about? Is there anything you need to vent about? Get it out. Sort through it. If you're unsettled with your provider, switch. (And go to step #2 below). If you realize that you are with your soul mate of a provider, woohoo! Celebrate!

2. Go online. Google OB/GYNs or Midwives in your area. If there are any negatives about those providers, you'll definitely find it online (check out RateMDs.com). As with anything online, take it with a grain of salt. *Of course you can't solely rely on "online info,"* but you'll learn a lot fast. And everything together adds up to a clear picture!

3. Do what Kate did: ask women with similar philosophies about birth and definitely ask your doula (or any doula-even if you decide not to use one) to connect you to providers in the area. They know *how* all the doctors or midwives interact with moms during birth. This alone could save you serious headache, stress, and wasted time starting out with the wrong provider.

4. Start interviewing them. Do this by phone or schedule interview appointments.

Take Action (continued)

If a provider isn't willing to meet with you for 15 minutes prior to hiring THEM to be your provider, then chances are, they probably aren't for you anyway (why would they listen to you down the road if they can't listen to you for a few short minutes now, ya know?)

5. Choose the one you feel the best fit with, the one whose approach to care is what you'd like.

Wow, mamas. You're crushin' this! Now let's go to lesson #4, the last one.

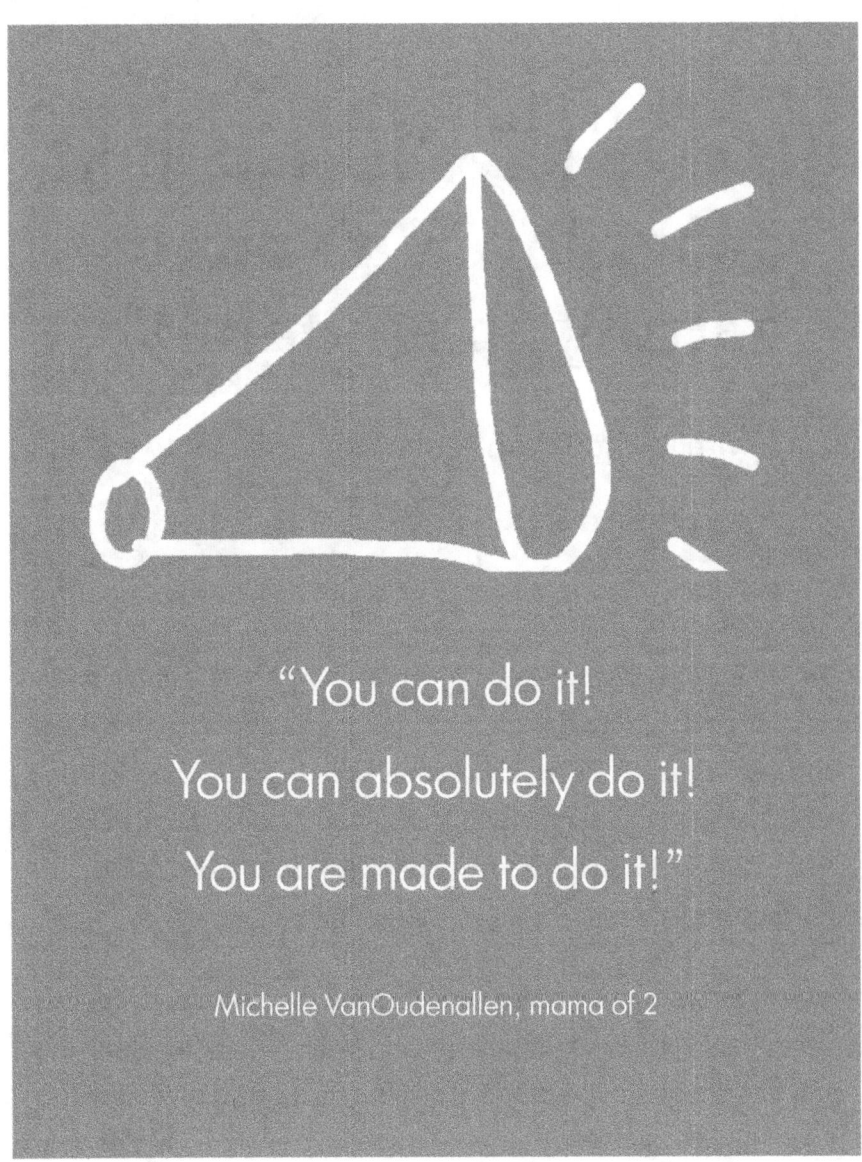

"You can do it!
You can absolutely do it!
You are made to do it!"

Michelle VanOudenallen, mama of 2

lesson four

"How to have less pain in labor {even if you're getting an epidural}"

-with Michelle VanOudenallen, mom of two girls

Sarah: How can you work through labor pain? There's going to be {some} pain in labor no matter what route you choose. Even if you plan on getting an epidural, sometimes they just don't work, don't work well, or you can't get one because you're labor goes so fast, etc. The point is...knowing how to deal with labor pain is *super* beneficial for any mama about to have a baby!

There are things that work really well, aside from drugs, that you can do to help cope with labor pain. So Michelle VanOudenallen is here to teach you how to deal super effectively with any labor pain you might have. She shares how to do it, gives examples, and even walks you through them.

She's the mother of two girls and she had two unmedicated births. Her first labor was 51 hours. I know you guys are all cringing, but she's going to teach you how she got through it (which she has a beautiful baby girl to show for), so you can get through any labor you might have! Her second birth was four hours.

What did you decide to do the first time around with Grey to prepare for birth?

Michelle: I really set the intention that I wanted to have a natural unmedicated vaginal birth and I really believe that the more you know and the more information that you have, the less fear you have going into the birthing process. I really think there are a lot of misconceptions going in, based on the way media portrays childbirth to look like. And most of the stories we hear tend to be negative.

And so, since I knew that I didn't want that, I had to go out and seek my own information. That's the first thing that I did. Then I enrolled in a HypnoBirthing class.

Sarah: Why did you do that?

Michelle: I wanted to be informed going in and I wanted to learn techniques and get myself a set of tools. I knew women got epidurals for a reason, and in order to avoid that, I knew there was going to be a level of pain that I was going to need to manage. And when push came to shove and I was in that place reconsidering an epidural or my body wanting medication...I wanted the mental tools, the emotional tools, and the reinforced ideas going in that would kind of keep me in the zone and in that original intention I set.

Sarah: Let's back track. We'll talk first about what specifically you did and what you learned in HypnoBirthing and then what helped you during each stage of labor. So what specifically did you learn in HypnoBirthing...what specific skills?

Michelle: The first thing I learned was a deep understanding of the different stages of labor. So when I was in those stages I *knew* that stage, I *knew* what to expect in that stage and therefore I *knew* how to cope with that stage without the fear of... "*is it going to get any worse? How long this is going to last?*" I had an understanding.

So when those unknowns were taken away, I was able to focus my mind on what was happening. So that's the first specific takeaway that helped me labor more easily.

Then once I was laboring, for example like in early labor, I took hot baths. The hydrotherapy was incredibly soothing. Some of the most helpful things were the kind of things that you want to do for yourself at the end of a really hard day. It's just self-care.

I wanted aroma-therapy. I lit candles. I put some bubbles in the bath, turned out the lights, and I just helped myself relax. Getting to a place of deep relaxation was really important for me and I think it's essential for any birthing mother or laboring mother, because when you are relaxed, your muscles are relaxed.

Your stress hormones aren't flying all over the place. You're in a better place to respond to what is going on. So those kinds of self-care principles are what I learned in the labor class and then I could use those at each stage.

Sarah: It sounds like you're going to have a tool box of options and things you can pick and choose from to see what works best for you?

Michelle: Absolutely.

Sarah: Did you practice these things before you gave birth? I know some childbirth classes really hammer that in... did you have it down before you actually needed it?

Michelle: Well I'm a certified yoga instructor and I've practiced meditation and taught meditation for relaxation, so I have some of those tools already. So yes, in that sense, I have been doing that for a long time.

Some of the specifics: they gave us a HypnoBirthing CD with scripts that they read, which were sort of deep relaxation exercises that I would play before I went to bed. I did that for months and actually I had it in the car on the way to the hospital birthing center, just because the familiarity of those were soothing to me. It helped kind of put me in that place of *"okay, this is what we're doing right now. We're getting ready to have the baby. This is what we have been practicing for."*

I also had some affirmations that I chose for myself. Certain affirmations addressed specific issues or fears that I had. Like, "my baby is the perfect size for my body" and I would just say that over and over again. Or I would envision my cervix being ready to open, then opening, and I would be breathing my baby down.

I was just envisioning the physiological changes that my body was going through as my body was changing, as I was giving birth. Instead of holding tightly, squeezing my muscles and thinking, *"oh my gosh, I don't what's going to happen, is this baby about to come out?"* I had the picture already happening in my head.

I pictured my hips widening. I pictured my cervix opening. I was picturing the birth canal just being open and smooth and ready for the baby. That is really helpful because it took away the unknowns of what was going to happen. I just went in knowing what's going on with my body.

Sarah: You mentioned that you used relaxation, affirmation, and some visualizing. Let's get back to the affirmation for a second, because I think a lot of people have fear about childbirth, which is really important to address beforehand. What do you recommend for people to do and how far in advance do people need to start thinking about it? Because there is kind of that fine line... you don't want to dwell on it but you also need to overcome it, so what's the balance there?

Michelle: Yeah, that's a great question, because I really don't advise women to begin thinking about birth—I don't start handing them my resources until they are really in their third trimester. You can use the affirmations for your pregnancy, but you don't want to start thinking about birth way early on.

You've got to focus on growing that baby and that's a whole different stage. But I do think your body starts to naturally prepare itself for labor.

I had to switch to a different practitioner and I had to say some affirmations to myself before I made that switch.

Like *"I'm in control of this situation"* and *"I'm in control of my body and the birth of my baby"*...I don't remember exactly what I said, but they're along those lines to help get me to that relaxed place.

I think sooner than later, but not too soon, if that makes sense? Second trimester I think is a good time, when you're really focusing on birth and as you get closer to the actual labor time when you'll be using them repeatedly.

Sarah: Okay, because obviously you want to remember what the affirmations are, so repetition is good to help you remember what to say that will actually get you to relax.

Michelle: Write them down and I wouldn't pick more than three. You don't want to have all these things that you've memorized, but they'll come to you. You know what fits you.

For me, just because I'm small and I had an experience when I was in middle school where some girl came up to me and said *"oh, you are going to have c-sections, you are so little."* Just out of the blue that came back and was in my head, so when I said, *"my baby is the perfect size for my body,"* that was *really* important to me. That girl randomly planted that lie at a really early age, the thing is we have so many lies and misconceptions we constantly tell ourselves that we don't even realize.

I mean, that was in seventh grade, we weren't even talking about babies. So those things are in our minds and identifying what they are and exposing them is a huge step to overcoming the fear they might bring along. You have to identify what you're afraid of and sometimes you don't even know what it is you're afraid of until you visualize what you'll be doing.

Sarah: So through your labor, your 51-hour labor with Grey, obviously when you're starting labor you don't know how long it is going to take, but you still have to prepare mentally the best you can. You said in early labor you were doing the hydrotherapy, the hot baths, things like that...as you progressed into active labor, what things were working for you best?

Michelle: Once I was in active labor, the hydrotherapy still... getting in a shower and really feeling the heat on my back, the counter pressure my husband or the midwife or the nurse was, I had a lot of back pain because she was in a posterior position. I felt I had to keep moving. I was swaying a lot. If I was feeling a surge, I didn't want to sink into it and I didn't want to give into it. So if I moved, it was almost like I was kind of just like fleeing for a moment—like I was keeping it fluid.

As I mentioned before, as soon as I was active labor, I was naked, like buck naked, and there was a reason for that. Not only because you're in and out of the shower, and you know what's funny, I had been, before birth, a moderately modest person...no longer is that the case. I'll take my shirt off right now!

Sarah: Yeah, show us, Michelle, show us what you really mean!

Michelle: One of the things that I learned in the HypnoBirthing class, it's so essential for a woman to be in a primal state. That includes not wearing clothes. I had to sort of strip civilization off of me. The same way you strip the media's "fear-based" images off of you, you have to really strip down, because birth is so core to our existence. It is a primal thing.

Women have been getting pregnant and giving birth forever, ya know? That's how the human race has been going on. And that's another affirmation that I said over and over, *"women have done this for thousands and thousands of years. I am one of the women who have done this for thousands and thousands of years,"* and I kept picturing early Native American women in red tents and all kinds of women throughout history in all kinds of crazy places. I mean women give birth all the time in a non-civilized environment, so I felt like that was huge... being naked and being primal, because when you go there, you can access some primal tools that you can't access otherwise.

Sarah: As labor was going on, when did you hit a wall? And if you did, how did you overcome that wall?

Michelle: I absolutely hit a couple of walls. One was sheer exhaustion, because I had labored for 12 hours at home and was just kind of doing stuff during the day. But I hadn't slept and you know, towards the end, you don't sleep too much anyway, so you know when I was going on 24 hours, I would fall asleep, have a contraction, then wake up. I didn't choose to do this, but one thing I would recommend for women who are beginning to hit the sleep deprivation wall, just remove all clocks and all sense of time from your birthing space. Because one of my fears was having a time frame imposed on me.

So if you don't know what time it is, it helps. I had no idea during labor that I was 7 cm dilated for 7 hours. It felt like 45 minutes. I had no idea. You definitely lose your sense of time, which is really good. One of the things that I did during that time was to kind of create sleep for myself. I'd still be laboring and doing the work of laboring, but it helped. There is a tool called sleep breathing.

Sleep breathing essentially is kind of tricking your body into deep relaxation by mimicking the kind of breathing that you do in sleep. So when you're sleeping, your breath tends to be really evened out, it tends to be really rhythmic, and it's like you're not really thinking about your breathing. You're letting your body just do its natural thing to get itself into a natural state of relaxation that ends up leading you to sleep. And so, you can create that by intentionally breathing that way and your body will automatically respond to that signal from your deep breaths and go into deep relaxation mode.

Sarah: It's kind of like you're pretending?

Michelle: Yes, exactly. It's like you're pretending to sleep. You're breathing, but you're pretending to sleep. So I'll just do a little demo. If I want to sleep, I'll close my eyes and I'm just going to do this for a few minutes or few seconds. (Does the demo with closed eyes—breathing slowly and deeply in and out.)

So if you were looking at me, you were thinking that I was either narcoleptic or that I had just fallen asleep, right? And really that's what you should look like.

It should look like you're asleep to others, because you're pretending to sleep and it's an incredibly effective method not only for relaxing your body, but to also get you centered. If you're focusing on your breath, you're only focusing on one thing, as opposed to all the stimulus around you, any discomfort you might be experiencing, any anxiety that might be creeping in. Continue to focus on pretending to sleep. That really, really made a huge difference.

Sarah: Because also when you're *pretending*, you're not focusing on how to do it a "right way" or a "wrong way"…you're just doing what works. And everyone can pretend, right?

Michelle: That's an excellent point! When you're pretending, you're sort of letting go of expectations you put on yourself or expectations that you read you should do or should be doing. You're in the moment, for one, and you're engaging in your right brain, which is playful and you don't really have any rules, and so that's exactly the kind of state you need to be in, to kind of slip into a primal state where you're able to just relax and let your instincts take over.

Sarah: What else did you do to kind of get over those walls?

Michelle: That was one reason I chose to give birth in a birthing center. I didn't want to feel that I was at all constrained by an IV or an epidural that would stop me from using my legs. I found that when I was moving, I was also actually moving around any discomfort. Movement prevented any nerves from being pushed for too long. So I did a lot of rocking, standing up and rocking—that was soooo helpful to me. And also rocking is really soothing, you know how babies liked to be rocked. That natural kind of moving the body back and forth to get soothed works and just feels really good in that moment.

At the very beginning of my labor, when those contractions were beginning, I would leave my room and do walks around the birthing center. When I was in the deep throws of active labor, I really liked squatting and I'd move back and forth.

I'd keep things moving so that I never focused on one kind of discomfort for too long. I also used a birthing ball, where I would sit on the ball with my legs like I was on a horse and it really felt amazing because it helped open up my pelvis. I would then sort of rock in that position, too.

Also it helps the baby in that positioning and helps get movement, so the baby isn't pressing on nerves during some of those contractions.

Sarah: You also mentioned distractions and distractions that you chose to have in the room with you?

Michelle: Yeah, totally. I think I mentioned I really wanted earplugs, because I thought if someone talked I was going to have another contraction. So no one spoke. There was no one in my birthing room talking. Even the nurses knew to keep it down.

So I did have earplugs in—I learned that the hard way the first time around, where noise was such a distraction for me. So my second birth, I brought earplugs with me—several pairs.

That was huge, because I felt like anything that was going to take my attention was going to keep me from focusing on the work that I needed to be doing. And it's work. It's like if you're writing a term paper or you're working on your dissertation, you don't want all kinds of random sounds or you won't be able to focus.

I also used music, and for me, music without words was essential. I had really low-key spa type music. I think mine was like Native American flute. But just something, it's whatever is soothing for you. I know other friends made birthing exercise music, like Justin Timberlake stuff.

It's not for me, but yeah, I do recommend bringing in creature comforts and things that are soothing. Kind of like when you're going on an airplane, you pack your little neck wraps and your iPod and all these little things to keep you comfortable during that uncomfortable time. I think you need to think about birthing the same way.

Sarah: You also mentioned that when you started hitting the wall you had a little pep talk with yourself in the bathroom. You had some alone time, what was that about?

Michelle: Well, I used the bathroom as that *"I need a minute…"* checkout time to go in and just get away from everyone. Because the bathroom is a place where you can lock the door, it just gives you a little space when you want it. And so I was in there a lot, not necessarily using the bathroom, but using the space.

There was a mirror in there and I would give myself pep talks, but before that, I had to have little reality checks with myself. Like I remember specifically looking in the mirror and saying, "*What are you thinking? Why did you choose to do this naturally again? You know the regular hospital is just 100 yards away, so if you want to go and do this the western medicine way, it's still available.*"

And I looked at myself and my hair was all over my face. It was all wet and I was like, "*You don't look very good. You are definitely going to need to put some makeup on, before the post-baby pics.*"

But I definitely used that time to check in with myself. Even those kinds of conversations and even looking at myself in that way was really helpful, because it brought me back to "*okay, let's go, this is you, you've been doing this, hello Michelle, you know you can do this!*"

I had to touch base with myself in that way... looking at myself in the mirror and sort of being like... "*hey, you are birthing right now... you are in it... you're doing this!*"

It's that moment you so look so forward to. It may not be "comfortable," but there's nothing more amazing or another time in your entire life where you're more in the moment. I feel like that was really important for me, even just being present and remembering what was happening.

I know lot of people that look back on their births and it's just a fog. It's like your wedding day, so much was going on. And I remember those moments with myself and they were really sacred, because I was choosing to sort of stop and be like, "*okay, this is what's going on, you're 7 cm dilated and you know you're getting ready to push! You gotta gear up, you gotta do this!*"

I also had a very significant moment that I remember right before I had Ingrid, my second baby. I remembered what crowning felt like and I was afraid I was going to tear, because I tore with my first baby. Looking back, it really wasn't that bad, but I just didn't want that to happen, so I remember even saying to my midwife that I wanted an episiotomy.

That's when you knew I was going through transition. If you know me at all, I am like the poster child for no episiotomies. She actually just started laughing at me in the middle of me saying I wanted one and my husband is going *"no no no!"* That's when I knew … *"okay, I'm getting close, because I'm not making any sense."* I didn't have an episiotomy, and I didn't tear, and it was awesome!

Sarah: Toilet sitting was really helpful for you, tell us about that.

Michelle: Back to the bathroom…

Toilet sitting is so huge. That is one of the single most effective ways of getting your body to relax and open up in "those regions."

Because the toilet is where you naturally open and release things, your body knows that. It doesn't open up like that walking down the street and it certainly doesn't open up in front of other people. So you're in a birthing center room with strangers around, your husband, and even if mentally you're okay with it, you haven't trained that lower part of your body to be okay with letting things out in front of others.

So when you sit on a toilet, Ina May Gaskin, one of the amazing spiritual midwives of our century, talks about sphincters, which are those things that open and close. They are shy, and so sitting on the toilet is sort of like warming them up and telling them like... *"hey, it's okay."* So I would sit there for extended periods of time holding my pillow. I like to reiterate in all my classes I teach how buck naked I was ... just to make that clear.

So I'm totally naked, I'm sitting on the toilet, I'm holding the pillow and I would just sort of do the sleep breathing on the toilet, but first it's amazing because that position is sort of preparing you, like your baby is kind of like *"okay, birth canal... we can kind of start scootin' that baby down."* And then also, it's giving your sphincters permission to do what they need to do.

So it was huge. It helped to loosen up all the muscles down there, because we hold all of those in tight when we're afraid. Tightening those muscles turns into a natural cause of pain, so if you can get those relaxed, you won't feel as much discomfort in that area.

Sarah: That makes so much sense, because when I think about going camping and trying to go to the bathroom in the woods, it doesn't happen very easily because our body isn't used to doing that, it's not in relax mode. But give me a toilet in the woods... I'm good. That makes a lot of sense!

Michelle: And we really have to take it into account, because birth is such a primal experience. It really wasn't intended to be so much around people, around white walls, medicine, and stuff, it was more of an in the woods experience back in the day and especially when medicine wasn't available.

Getting in that primal state lets your body do a lot of the work for you. It remembers. It knows exactly what to do.

Sarah: You also mentioned urinating hourly. Why is that helpful to overcoming the wall?

Michelle: That actually was something my midwife encouraged me to do, even if I didn't feel like it. And I'll tell you a lot of times I didn't feel like going pee. But it does relieve a lot of pressure and that's because the contractions alone are moving and pushing, and so if there is pressure inside your abdomen, you can sort of release it. It's definitely going to make a difference. It's kind of like when you have menstrual cramps and then you go to the bathroom and it kind of helps a little bit... it's the same thing. You're just creating space so that movement isn't pushing up against anything and that alone relieves discomfort.

Sarah: Good ninja tip, I like that. Let's go back to pep talks in the bathroom for a second. Setting short term goals, I know, for a lot of people, is another great technique that people use. Did you use these short term goals?

Michelle: Absolutely. I was sort of trained as an athlete when I would run. It was like, *"okay, if you can just make it to the mail box, if you can just make it to whatever,"* so that sort of definitely is in my psyche as far how I work. And I think that's just an effective tool no matter what your goal is, but particularly when you're so focused on your body and sometimes your body is trying to win out over your mind. When you can give your mind a task like that, it definitely helps it stay calm.

And the goal is to keep your mind calm and still so your body can do what it needs to do without any interference. You've got to just focus on the contraction. You know it's just... *"let's get through this."*

And I did, I did slip into that a lot, because especially when you've given birth before, it's a lot easier to jump ahead, because you know exactly what's coming up. But also when you have a goal, there is some determination that comes in and your fierceness shows up. If you're a competitive person, there is just sort of like *"I am going to beat my goal."* I was so excited when they filled up the tub for me for my second birth, I spent hours in the tub when I birthed Grey, my first, and this one, they filled it up, I got in for ten minutes, I got out and was like *"okay, done with the water."* I was so excited or something, I didn't even need the water, I was like *"I'm out!"*

Sarah: So it could be something as simple as saying *"I'm going to get through the next contraction or I'm going to get through the next time until my midwife comes back in or the nurse comes back in and checks me?"* I'm setting really short goals that are just right around the corner, maybe in the next 30 seconds or even a minute?

Michelle: Yep, exactly! I remember in the very end, during some of the pushing, my goal was my husband just coming back with some water! You know when those things happen and you're like *"I'm so thirsty"*... then all of a sudden all of your needs are crazy amplified? Well at first, for me, I was just thirsty, and then all a sudden I was dying of thirst.

So I remember having a little goal to just get through until the water comes in. And that was my reward. Or maybe it's the popsicle or whatever else for you.

Sarah: Let's talk about pushing for a second. What were the main things for both your labors that really helped you with the pushing?

Michelle: For one, my birth vision or birth plans that I gave my midwife showed that I wanted to do self-directed pushing. You know how the media or in movies, it's usually a doctor at the bottom end of a woman saying *"push, push, push"* and a woman just responds to that command. Not in my world.

So really it was... I would say *"I'm ready to push"* and when I'm ready to push, they would say... *"okay."* I don't really feel like the word pushing is accurate because it's not as much pushing as sort of this bearing down and helping something get out.

It's kind of like bearing down. Then you're using your muscles and you're pushing... okay, I guess you are pushing.

But I found pushing to be incredibly exhilarating, actually. You're so aware that you're in the final moments and your adrenaline is going and everything comes together. It's the part of my birth that I remember the most and with the most detail!

Sarah: You mentioned that trusting your body was really important. Why was that important for you during the pushing part?

Michelle: Because that's the scariest part and having knowledge about how my body works during the pushing was a relief for me. It relieved fear. So I knew, for example, that when the baby's head was going to be coming through the birth canal, the top of her head was going to be pressing on some of the nerves in my birth canal that was actually going to relieve some pain.

It was going to cut off some nerves and I knew that, and so knowing that, I thought… *"okay, that's a relief, I can trust that, that's going to happen. That's something I know is designed to happen."* I can handle that and you know because I was breathing my baby down, I was breathing and bearing down and I was ready to push… you get to the point that you want to push, because it feels good to push and so I knew that I was there. I knew no one else was telling me something to do that I wasn't ready to do. And that was really important.

My second birth I was super excited to get that baby out. I had been pregnant for like two years and I was having these babies so close together and was thinking, *"I am so ready to get this baby out of my body."*

That was a major motivation, too. When you've done it before, it went so much quicker because all my muscles remembered… they're like, *"oh… we're getting a baby out again… cool, we can do this."*

Sarah: You also mentioned that you had a relationship with your body prior to labor. What do you mean by that and how did that help you in labor?

Michelle: Absolutely, that's the part we go really, really deep inside. I mean, that's the part, like you said, I trusted my body, I let it go, like on auto pilot and let it do what it needed to do and that's where my eyes were absolutely closed. The room was absolutely dark. No one said a sound except if it was to guide me in one way or another for safety, or the baby.

My first birth, I had all my hair in front of my face. I looked like "IT" from the Adam's Family TV show and I felt like this cavewoman and it was awesome.

Sarah: It sounds like you were in the zone?

Michelle: I was in the zone. But in order to get in the zone, I had to, let me say one more time, be naked. And I mean get to the point where I stripped away anything that was of my "normal life," things I normally cared about, like how I looked—any of that. I just became a primal body.

You know I'm not trying to sound too hippie. I *really* believe in this, because birth is just one of those things ...you don't take a shower with your clothes on.

And you don't have sex with your clothes on, either. You know, it's in a way, one of those kinds of things that should just be you, naked, in the zone.

You should be so far in the zone that you don't care if you're naked... that's what I'm trying to say. You don't care because you're in your own deep, deep place and that's with the breathing and eyes closed and basically shutting off anything else around you.

Sarah: What advice do you have for mamas who are checking out the whole going natural vaginal childbirth thing? They may not know if they're gonna go with or without meds, but what advice do you give moms right now?

Michelle: Absolutely, I would say first of all... you can do it! You can absolutely do it! You are made to do it! Your body is designed to do it. You can, and if you choose not to, that's a choice, but I would say gather as much information as you can about the benefits of natural birth and medicated birth.

But don't make decisions by default and don't do it in ignorance.

So make sure you know what's going on, and what I found, when I weighed the knowledge and the evidence, natural made more intellectual sense to me. I felt safer about choosing to do a birth this way. It just felt better for me all around, for my body, and I wasn't afraid. I was more afraid of going into birth having my body constrained with all kinds of machines and then feeling constrained and just not having freedom to move. Freedom is really important to me and it's something that I value. I think that you need to bring your core values in your birthing experience, whatever those are for you.

Sarah: "Whatever those are for you" is a great place to leave it. There isn't one right way to have a baby, but there is definitely a right way for you. But you'll only know what that is by getting evidence-based information and asking a lot of questions! Knowledge trumps fear.

Supporting Evidence

Michelle talks a lot about being able to move around to relieve pressure, minimize pain, and work through labor. A growing amount of evidence is clear—women should labor and birth however is comfy for them.

The US Cochrane Center at the Johns Hopkins Bloomberg School of Public Health, reviewed 22 studies involving 7,280 women and concluded[viii]... *"women should be encouraged to give birth in comfortable positions, which are usually upright."*

But why and what do the benefits mean to you?

Your uterus is made up of muscles. Muscles are fueled by oxygen. Blood delivers that oxygen. When you have freedom to move around, more blood flow delivers more oxygen to your uterus. That means your uterine muscles work better and way more efficiently during contractions. More efficient contractions mean a faster labor and less pain, because your uterine muscles get more done in less time (ie—you get more bang for your buck with each contraction).

Ever pulled a leg muscle? What feels better: laying down in bed or standing up and moving around so your muscles get more blood flow and oxygen? Doesn't moving around feel like a gazillion times better? Same idea.

Movement also helps your sacrum (the large triangular bone sitting right at your pelvic opening) move in six different ways. And that allows your pelvis to open up as much as 30% more. A bigger opening gives your baby a lot more room to travel (easier and faster) through the birth canal. Yes, please.

In upright positions, your cervix dilates faster (baby's weight helps to open your cervix) and prevents you from having to push against gravity (like you would if lying down). You save energy and avoid your muscles working as hard. It's easier (for most women).

More oxygen gets to your baby because of the better positioning of the heart's large artery called the "descending aorta."

Most women in the US give birth lying on their back. According to the best medical research and evidence (and to most women who've given birth both ways... on their back and in various positions) ...giving birth on your back is the most painful way to give birth.

The takeaway is that the medical evidence supports you laboring and birthing in the positions that are most comfortable for you!

Michelle also talked about media doing a disservice to women. This study[ix] analyzed 85 reality-based tv shows showing 123 births and concluded *"this research suggests that reality-based birth television programs do not give women an accurate portrayal of how women typically experience birth in the United States, nor are the shows consistent with evidence-based maternity practices."*

No big surprise, right? TV networks' focus is on making money, not educating women with the best evidence-based maternity care. They make more money by sensationalizing birth, because it gets more people watching, which brings in more advertising dollars. TV networks' loyalty is to their shareholders, not to you and your baby.

In Short

Steve and I took a pretty typical birth class prior to our son being born. If you would have asked me at the time how it was, I would have told you "great."

In retrospect, it wasn't.

The reason it wasn't helpful was because we weren't taught all our options. We were told things like *"when you get an epidural, you will..."* but there wasn't talk of how to cope with pain or what other pain medication options besides an epidural there are. It was kind of like showing up to a restaurant, and instead of helping us understand all our delicious options, we were given a set menu and told this is what you'll have and this is how it'll taste. It's like our meal had already been chosen for us. After our class, we found out that we had soooooo many more options than we ever knew about. Birth class fail.

Thankfully, I armed myself with a bit of extra knowledge so that I had extra tools during labor to help me.

I learned the hard way why choosing the right provider is critical, because having candid, awesome, honest conversations with my doctor beforehand helped us be on the same page about how we really wanted our birth to go down (so to speak).

I also learned that if you choose to give birth in a hospital, the nursing staff can be a wild card. So learning how to communicate your wishes without being perceived as obnoxious and snooty is KEY.

A great example is our friend Jamie was laboring with her first baby. At one point she had been pushing for three hours and her doctor suggested they get ready for a c-section since baby wasn't crowning yet. Jamie calmly and confidently asked, *"how's my baby's heart rate?"* They responded that it was fine. She asked, *"how's my blood pressure?"* They said, *"good."* And her last question was *"do I have a fever or anything?"* they responded, *"No."* Then Jamie responded, *"If I'm fine and the baby's fine, why are you suggesting a c-section?"*

The doctor agreed to give her more time to let her body do what it was meant to do. After five hours of pushing, her baby was born vaginally. Woohoo! This is a great example of asking probing questions, but in a manner which was not threatening or know-it-all-like. It was just conversational. And confident.

She took the info she was given by her provider, matched it with the info she knew about birth, herself, and her body... then TOGETHER came to a decision (with her provider). They were a team. Teams usually make the best decisions.

As I wrote in my book, Going to the MotherLand, my doula (or birth Sherpa as my husband likes to call her) was like my Swiss Army Knife secret weapon. She was the one who gave me great ideas that got me the best results to keep labor progressing. One of the BEST suggestions she gave was one that Michele mentioned: hydrotherapy.

1-Hydrotherapy is just a fancy name for water therapy. For all the same reasons swimming is so good for our body and taking baths is relaxing, it's also good for labor. It helps your contracting uterine muscles work super efficiently. A study including 3,243 women showed how many women didn't even request pain medication and had more "satisfaction" with their birth experience. You can use hydrotherapy in labor or just to birth your baby or both.

The hospital where I gave birth didn't have birth tubs, so I took my birthing ball into the shower and sat on it while warm water ran down my back. The warm water hitting my lower back and sitting on the ball relieved a ton of pressure and helped me stay calmly focused. I stayed in there forever. Ask Steve, he was about to pass out from the steam sauna I had going on. It was heavenly!

The other comfort measures that Michele mentioned are:

2-Affirmations—positive truths that you want to remember or repeat to yourself during labor. Your body follows your mind. That's why top athletes use them all the time (and tons of other high performing peeps)! People get better results when they affirm to themselves where they're going. It works. It's proven. The better result in my second birth was relaxation. I kept reminding myself to "open up." That helped me not tense my muscles. *I was a lot more relaxed in my second birth using affirmations than I was in my first when I didn't use the "open up" affirmation.*

3-Short term goals—help you get over the hump during labor. Set achievable short goals so you feel a lot of "small victories." After a small victory, you start believing more in yourself. Then you start affirming yourself more. "I'm doing it, I can do it, I'm doing it, I can do it, I'm closer to meeting my baby!" Next thing you know, you'll be holding your baby! Whoo hoo!

4-Sleep breathing—pretending to sleep by breathing deeply (like you are sleeping) tricks your body into relaxing. By consciously breathing slowly and deeply, your brain sends signals telling your body to relax—this lowers your blood pressure, decreases your heart rate, and helps you stay focused on meeting your baby. Try it, it works! I'm relaxed right now!!

5-Toilet sitting—I know, I know, most of us don't associate anything toilet-related with birth... but it's *all* in your mind. And that's exactly why it works (remember, your body follows your mind). Your upper leg muscles are supported, gravity works in your favor and your pelvic floor relaxes. Our mind is conditioned to relax and "let it out" when we're on the toilet. And the same applies when in labor. Trust millions of moms who swear by it. Try it during your labor and just see if it helps you progress faster and manage contractions more easily. Who knows, it could be *the best* suggestion anyone ever gave you for labor. No biggie if it doesn't work, but at least you tried. For a lot of women, magic just happens when you sit on the toilet during labor.

6-Pep talks—similar to affirmations, pep talks are where you just have a sit down with yourself and remind yourself where you are and what you're doing—a great way to instantly refocus on your baby from any distraction.

7-Counter pressure—having your labor support press on your back relieves pain (for every mama we've talked to) as baby makes its way through the birth canal. Lightly rolling a tennis ball is super helpful, or just pressing with the hand also relieves pressure.

8-Music—soothing music or rock music may help you get into a "labor rhythm" of breathing, pushing, or making progress towards meeting your baby. It also helps you create your own space within a hospital or birth center. Remember from the Dr. Fischbein class how the environment around you is proven to increase your chances of going into labor naturally, decreasing the need for interventions, improving birth satisfaction, etc. It works.

9-Going to the bathroom—Because your uterus sits right on top of your bladder, emptying your bladder creates more space for baby to move on down the birth canal. It's also a great way to get some privacy and quiet if you want to refocus with a pep talk (especially if you feel like everyone is just watching you).

10-Get naked (both literally and figuratively). Get to work by getting into the zone—this may mean losing your clothes (if that suits you). Stripping off expectations and distractions can help you go where you need to go (internally). And if you want to go to that place (wherever it is for you), but can't find a way to get there, sometimes just physically doing something gives your mind the permission it was waiting for... and away you go. *Motion creates the emotion to get you there.* This might mean facing some of your fears early on in your pregnancy. Writing them down, then letting them go will help you speed up labor.

11-Breathe—it sounds like a "duh." But remembering to breathe, finding a rhythm with your breath, and feeling the freedom to breathe however you want and need, to relieve pain. Focusing so much on "breathing right" can be counter-productive and work you into a frenzy (because you feel like you're doing it all wrong). There is no "perfect" or "right way" to breathe. Breathe however is most comfortable for you.

Take Action

1. What was one thing Michelle said that struck a chord with you? (Whatever it is...write about it right now in your journal for 3 minutes...just write.)

2. Which 3 of the "comfort measures" listed above do you want to learn more about (even if you plan on getting an epidural)? These are super important to learn. Sometimes epidurals don't work or just partially work...knowing these makes sure you're ready for either during labor.

Where do I go from here?

So where do you go from here? What do you do with this treasure trove of information you've learned? We have a motto at Your Baby Booty: *"There's no one right way to birth a baby, but there's a right way for you."* I think that pretty accurately describes where you go from here, but only you will find what that is.

Maybe it means starting the interview process, or as I like to call it, "dating your doctor or midwife." Perhaps it's breaking up with your provider and finding your soul mate, even if you are in your third trimester and about to pop (yes, you can do that!).

It could mean you're just going to relax for a while, maybe in a super cozy warm bath (with hubby bringing you grapes and some delicious cheese), and doing nothing except soaking up all the lessons and experience others have shared, then filing them away for next time.

You could simply start asking "why" or "what evidence supports that recommendation?" when your provider suggests something you aren't too sure about.

Or just revel in the bliss of having a provider whom you trust and who sits with you on the floor while you're in labor.

You might decide to write a five word affirmation that you know makes you feel strong or notecards of the pain management techniques Michelle shared (so you can flip through them in 30 seconds, twice a week, so you'll remember them when you're in labor).

Do. Something. Small actions will give you BIG results. Even just a little tiny action that takes you one small step closer towards your goal builds momentum. Then comes confidence. It snowballs.

Congrats!! ...Awesome job! You're done reading this book!! Well, almost done...

Take 1 minute...

Grab your journal. Take 1 minute and write down the one thing you want to do after reading this book. Make one of those check mark boxes next to it. When you're done doing that 1 item, cross it off your list. Ahhhh. Doesn't that feel good?

Final thoughts...

Hi friend! We hope you enjoyed reading as much as we enjoyed writing this book.

Wherever you are in your journey, remember there are millions of women who have gone before you who had apprehensions just like you (I'm one of them), and have done it. It's normal. It's okay.

You can do it, too. You can!

You were made to do this, wherever and however you choose. It's pretty cool that we women with children share a common bond of perseverance, of strength, of digging deep and seeing parts of ourselves we never thought we'd see.

The journey to the MotherLand is one amazing ride. Challenging for sure. But well worth every second when you meet your baby and fall in love. Just remember... even when you feel like you can't...you can do it. You are doing it!

Our love to ya,

Sarah & Steve

*Can we ask a favor? If you liked the book, it'd mean the world to us if you'd use 2 minutes to write a quick Amazon review sharing how & why this book helped you. We've worked hard to bring you a book that would impact your pregnancy & birth- your review would *really* help Birth Book reach more moms during pregnancy and* birth. The review is easy and fast to do (it literally takes just a few minutes)...

1. Go to Amazon.com and type in "Birth Book #1", then click on the book title.
2. Click "Customer Reviews"(it's below the title, next to the stars & in-between the parenthesis)
3. Click on the "Create your own review" button (on the left side).That's it!

Thank you so much, we're very grateful! ☺

Thank You!

Walking along your journey to the motherland can be lonely, tiring, super exciting, fun, frustrating, and at times, boring. You're tirelessly devoted to your kiddos, yourselves, and your families. Sharing one tiny little bitty part of your journey with you is a big honor! So thank you!

And super special thanks to Dr. Hays, Dr. Fischbein, Michelle, and Kate! Learning from all your experience, honesty and insights is so helpful- thanks for sharing your wisdom! Thank you to our amazing community of moms at Your Baby Booty for inspiring us to do this work. We love serving you and helping you any way we can. Thanks also to all the mamas who helped us edit (read: "chopped") this book to make it better for you. We love ya'll and are so grateful!

If you liked this book...

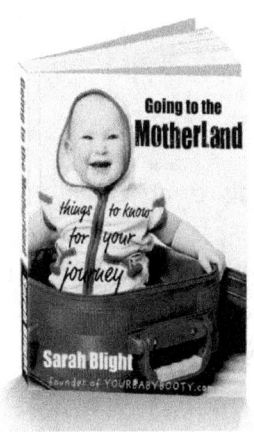

Pick up Sarah's first book, "Going to the MotherLand: things to know for your journey."

"Going to the MotherLand" is the honest-to-goodness, uncensored scoop about a first-time mama's journey through conception, raging hormones, pregnancy woes, getting baby out and figuring out what the hell to do next. Written for real moms with real questions, reading this book feels more like you're chatting it up with your best friend (with favorite beverage in hand) than reading a "pregnancy and childbirth book."

Carrie said *"Such a great read for anyone planning a journey to the new and strange land of parenting. It's filled with hilarious commentary, combined with honest and well-researched dialogue about pregnancy, birth, and the postpartum period. I wish this book had been on my shelf for babies #1 and #2. Maybe it'll inspire me to try for #3!"*

Natalie said *"Every mom should read this book! She had me laughing throughout! Easy to read and educational! Highly recommended to many friends already!"*

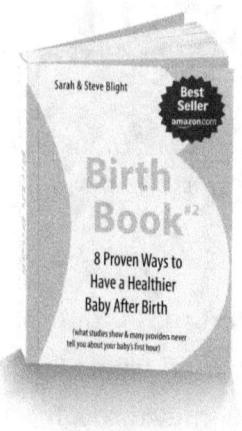

Our newest Birth Book is now available! Birth Book #2: 8 Proven Ways to Have a Healthier Baby After Birth (what studies show & many providers never tell you about baby's first hour)

The best hospitals, doctors, midwives and researchers know there are scientifically proven ways you can improve your baby's health during the most critical hour of their life, their first hour.

But most providers and birth classes never tell you what these are.

If our babies miss out on these benefits, they're missing out on critical health boosts that affect healthy brain development, how well their vital organs work, how strong their immune systems will be to fight off nasty infections, and lots more.

You deserve to know what these are, so your baby can get the benefits too!

We've asked some of the best and most sought after doctors, midwives and researchers in the world to teach you exactly what these benefits are and how to get them for your baby.

You'll learn:
-How to help your baby breathe easier & avoid respiratory distress
-How to help you baby avoid anemia (10x lower chance says Dr. Alan Greene)
-How to easily give your baby up to 33% more iron rich, oxygen rich & stem cell rich blood
-How to strengthen your baby's immune system ... and a lot more.

All our books are available on Amazon.com.

If you'd like to get an email when we release our next new book, just drop your email here to

www.yourbabybooty.com/ybb/future-books

Or just say hi, I'd love to hear from you! Email me at
Sarah@yourbabybooty.com

Copyright

Sources

---

[i]

http://www.ncbi.nlm.nih.gov/pmc/articles/PMC1948093/#citeref1
4

[ii] http://summaries.cochrane.org/CD003766/continuous-support-for-women-during-childbirth

[iii] http://www.ncbi.nlm.nih.gov/pubmed/2013951/

[iv] http://summaries.cochrane.org/CD000012/alternative-versus-conventional-institutional-settings-for-birth

[v] http://yourbabybooty.com/resources-101/feeling-overwhelmed-or-have-any-fear-of-pregnancy-and-childbirth/

[vi] http://summaries.cochrane.org/CD003766/continuous-support-for-women-during-childbirth

[vii] http://yourbabybooty.com/interviews/how-my-emotions-controlled-my-labor-how-yours-will-too/

[viii] http://summaries.cochrane.org/CD002006/position-in-the-second-stage-of-labour-for-women-without-epidural-anaesthesia

[ix] http://www.ncbi.nlm.nih.gov/pubmed/20557536

www.ingramcontent.com/pod-product-compliance
Lightning Source LLC
Chambersburg PA
CBHW060405290526
45791CB00002B/615